NEW HORIZONS
AND
MY ANGELS

WRITTEN BY ACAYSHA

Printed in Victoria, Canada

acaysha@newhorizonsandmyangels.com
www.newhorizonsandmyangels.com

National Library of Canada Cataloguing in Publication

Acaysha
    New horizons & my angels / Acaysha.

ISBN 1-55369-459-7

    1. Acaysha. 2. Epileptics—United States—Biography. 3. Depressed persons—United States—Biography. 4. Cancer—Patients—United States—Biography. I. Title. II. Title: New horizons and my angels.

RZ440.A23 2002   362.1'96853'0092   C2002-901850-1

TRAFFORD

This book was published *on-demand* in cooperation with Trafford Publishing. On-demand publishing is a unique process and service of making a book available for retail sale to the public taking advantage of on-demand manufacturing and Internet marketing.
On-demand publishing includes promotions, retail sales, manufacturing, order fulfilment, accounting and collecting royalties on behalf of the author.

Suite 6E, 2333 Government St., Victoria, B.C. V8T 4P4, CANADA
Phone	250-383-6864	Toll-free	1-888-232-4444 (Canada & US)
Fax	250-383-6804	E-mail	sales@trafford.com
Website	www.trafford.com		

TRAFFORD PUBLISHING IS A DIVISION OF TRAFFORD HOLDINGS LTD.
Trafford Catalogue #02-0272   www.trafford.com/robots/02-0272.html

10   9   8   7   6   5   4   3   2

DEDICATION AND MANY THANKS

*I would like to dedicate this book to **Dr. Hirschorn and Dr. Zimmerman of the Scottsdale Mayo Clinic,** my neurologist and neurosurgeon, respectively, for making this new life and dream possible ! Thank you for giving me a chance at a better life. May this story touch many others and give them the courage to have the surgery and take a chance at a better life! You both are truly angels in disguise – thank you for touching my life !*

MANY THANKS

Many people have touched my life in the nine years that I have been writing this story. Thanks to each of you who asked along the way, "How's the book coming ?" Your interest and support has made this creation not only mine, but ours ! Thanks for helping to keep me focused on the end result and finishing this project so I can share it with the world. I would also like to thank all of my friends, too numerous to mention, for their unconditional love and support along this journey.

Also thanks to all of my spiritual teachers and healers who have come into my life and enriched it for the better. Thanks for all of the healings, guidance and teachings, I have received, I couldn't have done it without you!! Thank you to my **editor Merriam Joan "MJ" Handy, "The Joy Lady."** Without her expertise, this book would never have come to be.

Finally, I thank my family for the many years you stood beside as we waited and hoped for an end to this struggle and the beginning of a new and better life. May it lead us all toward a complete healing and rejuvenation for all of the struggles, heart - ache, pain and suffering we all endured, each in our own way.

Thanks mom and dad !!
I do love you !!

Here are a couple of pictures of me, from the beginning of this journey to the end. I am four years old and in my second year of epilepsy in the first picture and I am 34 years old, receiving my bachelor's degree and 9 years SEIZURE FREE in the second picture.

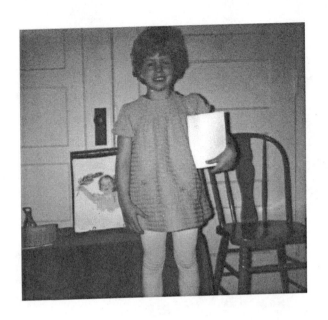

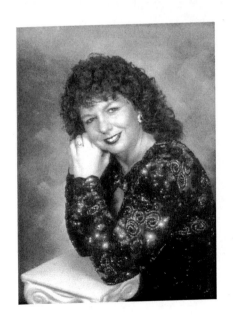

DEDICATION TO ACAYSHA

SOMEONE WHO IS CARING, FORGIVING,
KIND, THOUGHTFUL, GENEROUS, SPECIAL,
ANGELIC AND A TRUE FRIEND;
SOMEONE WHO HAS BEATEN THE ODDS
AND WAS REBORN;
SOMEONE WHO ACCEPTED CHALLENGES
WITH DIGNITY AND GRACE;
SOMEONE WHO WALKS ON **FAITH**;
SOMEONE WHO HAS TAUGHT ME TO
TAKE RISKS;
SOMEONE WHO LIVES LIFE TO THE
FULLEST;
SOMEONE WHO TOUCHES THE LIVES OF
MANY;
ALL OF THESE THINGS DESCRIBE - - -
ACAYSHA.

MANY BLESSINGS,

REV.KARAN WILKINSON

TABLE OF CONTENTS

THE BEGINNING OF A FANTASTIC JOURNEY – THE INTRODUCTION CHAPTER. 1

In a time when the world is in crisis, I have been guided to channel this book. Hopefully it will give people inspiration and hope in a time of tears and fears. As we all mourn the loses of many, we start to re-examine our lives and the meanings. So my book is meant to be an inspiration to all, whether you are fighting a major illness or dis-ease or you are just having a bad day. This book is meant to inspire and motivate you into giving yourself the strength to keep going and find new answers for your own life. I am hoping to help others move through their challenges and difficulties they face in this lifetime, and to inspire more epileptics to step out of their comfort zone and have the innovative, yet miraculous surgery I had and start living their lives ! Many epileptics are labeled handicapped, because people are scared of the attacks, but under that

scary surface is usually a wonderful
person, waiting to emerge.

You see, I have had many of my own
personal challenges and defeats to deal
with in this lifetime – starting with epilepsy
at the age of 2 and dealing with it for the
first 22 years of my life; going through
brain surgery and recovery; drowning in
depression and suicide thoughts; over -
coming migraines and uterine cancer -
with 6 months to live; to finishing college
with a bachelors degree in marketing –
graduating with honors, to being nine
years seizure free in 2001 and living life to
the fullest.

I started my life over almost 10
years ago (Oct 13, 1992) – when I decided
to conquer my epilepsy- after living with it
for over 22 years. On the average I had 3 -
5 seizures every month, which I thought
was *"normal,"* until I had 22 seizures in
less than 30 days and 6 anxiety attacks
that I had never had before. The anxiety
attacks scared me so badly that I ended up

in the emergency room everytime for 6 - 8 hours at a time – having Valium pumped into my veins in outrageous quantities to try to bring them to a halt. I finally decided I didn't want to fight this world alone anymore. My parents had moved 6000 miles away to England and I was finally scared.... **really scared !!** It took God 24 years to scare me.... and this time he/she surely did it !

      I called my mom after one of my "trips to the hospital" to tell her, *"I quit – I don't want to fight this world alone any – more !!" "I just want to come home and be your little girl"* were the words out of my mouth; words my family had **NEVER** heard me say before. You see, I was a fighter – I had experienced epilepsy since I was 2 years old, so I grew up with it - it was part of whom I was. I learned to deal with it, but it was also part of my hidden drive to ***"beat this world."***

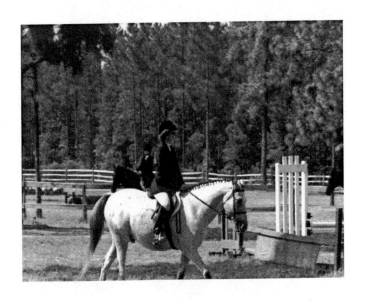

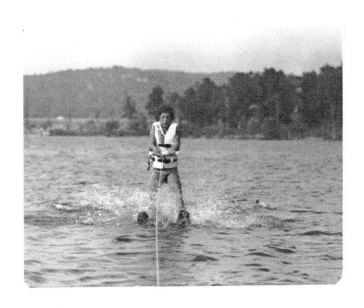

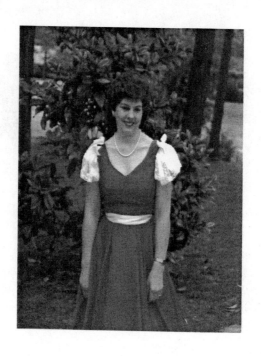

I was the ultimate poster child for epilepsy - nothing seemed to stop me. I drove cars, rode horses, did gymnastics, dated boys, moved away from home, went to college, moved 38 times in 35 years and graduated from college with an AA degree in 1988 in Retail Management / Buying / Merchandising – a specialized degree I have used in my career for over 13 years ! I now have my bachelor's degree in Marketing, which I received after nine years of pursuing it while going through brain surgery recovery !

You see my parents, especially my mom, raised me to strive to be *"normal"* and not let my epilepsy be a handicap or disease. I commend her for instilling that into me at an early age! She was so shocked by my quitting words that she quickly tried to comfort me, telling me that the seizures and anxiety attacks would calm down soon. She then suggested I call the Mayo Clinic and see if there was any new medications or techniques out there that we could try. Reluctantly, I agreed to call them. Since I had already tried every anti-seizure medication available on the market, and in every possible combination, I finally called the Mayo Clinic in Scottsdale Arizona, hoping to find some new answers to a very old problem. I was at my wits end and was ready to quit trying and fighting, prior to making this phone call.

Little did I realize how drastically my life would change, when I eagerly agreed to have this innovative surgical procedure done. I thought this was going to be the answer to all of my problems and an *EASY* way out of this life and into a *"perfect life."* (boy was I in for a surprise !) I was guided by God to go through with this new brain surgery, as it was going to be my answer to become epilepsy free and have a new life. I just wasn't informed how long and hard the recovery road was going to be !

This has been the hardest, most challenging, exciting, invigorating, frustrating, yet rewarding thing I have ever undertaken before in this lifetime.

To make this situation even more complex, my parents had returned to England for a new job assignment earlier that year and I had just started my cosmetic business so I was all alone, with my parents 6000 miles away and living on another continent ! In tackling the problems and obstacles that came, unforeseen by anyone, I have been through the dark -

est of days, scariest of moments and most rewarding of times, *all by myself.*

My mom flew back and forth constantly for the first year, trying to make the transition easier for me, but when my mom wasn't around, I was all alone to fend for myself and teach myself all about life. While she was there, she would do all the cooking, cleaning, laundry, etc.... she would *"just do it"* as the Nike commercial would say. Mom was definitely **an angel in disguise !**

Unfortunately that became her favorite phrase for everything in life.... *"you just do it !"* But to a 2 year old, the instructions on *"how to do laundry," "how to cook a meal" and "how to clean house"* aren't so simple and one technique doesn't do all those things. I wish it did ! I got quite frustrated to say the least and started asking other people questions on the *"how-to-do-it"* program of life. I had to re-learn everything - including washing my clothes, preparing a meal, scrubbing the bathroom etc. etc.!

I mentally and emotionally regressed back to the age of 2 – when my seizures first began and had to start from scratch learning everything all over again !! Have you ever let your 2-year-old be in charge of the family laundry, fix your meals or pay your bills ? Well I did it – even though I made many white clothes come out with pink spots, (because I didn't sort them from the reds,) and got all the "fuzzies" on my clothes from washing them with the towels !

I even burnt my first meal – pasta, black as the ace of spades ! The instruct - ions said add water to a pot and bring it to a boil – they didn't say how long it would take to make it boil. So I put the water on the stove, turned on the burner, and then walked away for almost 30 minutes ! I still had short-term memory loss at this time. Finally I returned to the kitchen and boy was it boiling ! The next direction said add *"desired amount of pasta."* What is a *"desired amount ?"* - **I was hungry so I put the whole box in !** Then it said to bring it back to a boil - **ugh !** Boy this takes forever to do, or at least I thought so ! So I went and played solitaire on my computer for almost 45 minutes ! At this point the smoke detector was going off and I didn't know what to do ! I ran into the kitchen and there was lots of smoke everywhere. **Scared, I called my mom in England,** asking *"is it done yet ?"* *Remember I was only 2, mentally and emotionally !* She was startled, as she could hear the smoke detector going off ! She then proceeded to tell me to open all the doors to let the smoke out. Then she told me to go put water in the pan, so I tried to pick up the hot pan without any hot pads or mitts, as she forgot to mention that. I jumped back and dropped the pan because it was burning my hands ! *Ouch !!* Realizing what happened she had me put it back on the stove and just bring

a glass of water to it. I did and it caused a lot of steam every –where ! Then I asked again, *"was it done ?"* as I was so hungry. She informed me that I had burnt the pasta and needed to just throw the entire pan away. I didn't understand !! So she told me this time to use hot pads and throw it in the trashcan, so I did – *water and all !* Swash went the water as it hit the bottom of the trash can ! Frustrated at this point, she asked me if I emptied the water out first, I said *"NO, you didn't tell me to !"* This is one of my favorite stories, as it shows you how much I had to learn all over again. I ended up having a sandwich, so I didn't have to cook anything ! After that, I learned it only took 8 minutes to bring the water to a boil and the entire meal was done in less than 15 minutes ! I ended up making pasta a major staple in my diet for almost 5 years ! *I love to cook now, but those beginning days were priceless !*

Luckily I learned quickly after doing something one time, whether right or wrong, because it was just like deja vous and I would remember just how to do it ! I went through puberty in 6 months, not 6 years like most youngsters ! I moved 15 times over that 10-year period, trying to find answers and people to help speed up my healing process. I yearned to *"be normal"* and healthy and was willing to do anything, move anywhere and try whatever was natural to get well !

My family, friends and myself were all very unprepared and ill-equipped to deal with all the challenges that I was destined to face, including massive depression, anger, migraine headaches, and suicide attempts. Through this process, I have become very spiritual and holistic and completely *"in tune"* to my body and its needs – learning natural ways of healing and feeling good. Little did I know this experience would benefit me personally and career wise in the future.

Going through all these changes and challenges, I was really very scared and overwhelmed; yet I didn't really know how to ask for help properly. So I would do dumb things to get attention like: drink lots of alcohol, which I had never done in my epileptic years; to trying to commit suicide by over-dosing on pills and medi – cations; and running away from home for days on end without telling anyone where I was ! I can now see this today as childish pranks and ways of getting attention, but coming through it I thought it was all the real thing and good options to choose !

I had a very strong will to survive the surgery and be successful, but I was also very unequipped to do the job by myself. I never realized how strong I was in dealing with the epilepsy all my life, from the age of two on, until I didn't have it anymore to lean on. You see seizures had their place in my life, as they were wonderful stress detectors. If I stressed out, I had a seizure and the level of stress would be reduced significantly. If I was too tired, not enough sleep, too hot, too cold, too emotional (good or bad) I had a seizure !! I walked a very straight and narrow line, trying to control my seizure activity.

Now, after surgery, the seizures were gone, so I had no coping tools or ways to deal with stress, exhaustion, poor diet, climate changes, etc. I had to re-develop or re-create my *"tool kit"* for life. These bi-polar swings were frustrating, exhausting and very overwhelming at times! I was definitely going through manic bi-polar swings and didn't even know it, until later ! If I stressed out too much, I would have an anxiety attack, a migraine headache or some form of a panic attack. These were my first skills I learned in my new tool kit for life. I have since replaced them with meditation, prayers, and visualization, herbs and exercise – *but many years later !!*

Having to re-learn everything, I have become the biggest book worm in the world, so I read all the time, attend seminars and listen to many tapes. I keep trying to understand the purpose of life, success, happiness, health and wealth – as all of these have the potential to be conquered in one lifetime !!

I have read every book and listened to every tape out there on portraying the *"right image;"* how to portray confidence in one's self; finding peace within while the world is chaotic; finding your *"real self"* and life's purpose; speaking with your angels and learning to love it; getting motivated and motivating others; and finding the blessing and good in every - thing. Through this great journey and all the stages of recovery of my new life, I have seen and experienced some very dark and dreary days; I have risen to the brightest of dawns; I have lived through gut-wrenching moments of great horror; and been awed by the greatest despair side-by-side with the greatest achieve -

ments and accomplishments one could ever experience !!

All of these extreme life experiences have benefited and prepared me to tackle today's obstacles and challenges. I have now learned never to give up, no matter how tough and trying it may get. I believe any goal I set is worth achieving, no matter how many big stone walls I have to climb over to get there ! Obstacles became my middle name for a while, because I was re-learning every aspect and phase of life. I tried many ways and techniques to learn, heal and grow and not all of them were easy and stress free. The *"boot camp training of life"* that I went through during the first six years of my recovery, which caught me back up to my physical age, were very trying times. It consisted of growing up, learning to cook again, finding the new *"me"* of myself, learning right from wrong, going to work, going to school, remembering how to play, and finding balance and love in my life.

Through this period of re-understanding the game of life, I have blossomed into a wonderful, dynamic, young lady, who knows who she is and where she is going. ***"Nothing is going to stop me now,"*** has become my mantra. My ultimate professional goal is to become a public speaker, (maybe even the female Zig Ziglar of the world.) not only for epileptics, but also for anyone trying to overcome an illness or disability, or for those feeling discouraged or depressed. I feel like I can conquer anything now with no limitations. *The sky is not even my limit !!*

I hope to inspire you, motivate you and delight you, leaving you counting your blessings each and every day ! I will share my newfound wisdom and life experiences with you as my wonderful team of angels continues to teach me new ways of living, laughing and loving. My angels have taught me so much about enjoying the journey we all call *"life."* I am now being guided to share that knowledge with you !

These and many more life-changing experiences will be shared with you in this true-life story ! ***ENJOY !!!***

IN THE BEGINNING...
THE DECIDING POINT - CHAPTER 2

In Late August 1992, I started to face the biggest challenge I had ever faced in 24 years. I needed to decide whether I wanted to keep living the way I had been living or change it dramatically. You see I had been an epileptic since I was 2 years old, and *3-5 seizures a month was "normal" to me*. But in the Fall of 1992, that activity jumped dramatically to **22 seizures in one month !** I was finally scared of them myself, and on top of that I was having anxiety attacks too.

These anxiety attacks looked like Grand Mal seizures, but they weren't, because I was conscience and could talk to people during them. Experiencing *22 seizures and 6 anxiety attacks in less than 30 days* scared me so badly, that I more than once I ended up in the emergency room. Each time, I was there for about 6 - 8 hours, having Valium pumped into my veins in magnificent quantities as the Doctors tried to bring the attacks to a halt.

Exhausted, I finally decided I was too frightened and too *"pooped"* to fight this world by myself anymore. My parents had moved across the waters to England and after 24 years of being a brave poster child, this time I really felt out of control. *For almost ¼ of a century I stood brave and unafraid, but before God, I was really scared this time !* During one of my hospital adventures, I decided to call my mom and told her *"NO MORE." "I QUIT."* I told her, ***"I don't want to fight this world alone anymore."*** These words were screaming out of my mouth – words my family had **NEVER** heard me say before and certainly not in such a desperate way.

I always prided myself in being a fighter. I grew up knowing epilepsy on a daily basis from the age of two...that was the *"me"* back then that I knew. I had learned to live with epilepsy; I had learned to live with being an epileptic child, but always inside me was a hidden drive to *"beat the epileptic world"* that forced me to be different from others. You see, no one could ever tell me, *"you can't do that; you're epileptic"* or *"you shouldn't do that because you might have a seizure."* Those were fighting words to me so I would just go do the opposite; I would go out and do whatever they said I couldn't or shouldn't do and do it faster and better than them, just because they lit my internal fighting fire !

I should have been on a telethon for epilepsy I was such a rarity, as nothing seemed to stop me. I learned to drive fast cars; I rode horses like the wind; I trained in gymnastics like I was trying out for the Olympics; I went to dances with boys; I showed-off my independence by moving out of the house; I braved the gruel of going to college; I very skillfully moved 38 times in 35 years; I even graduated from college with an AA degree in 1988 In Retail Management, Buying, and Merchandising.

This is a specialized degree I have used in the Image and Fashion world for over 13 years, and now have my bachelor's degree in marketing too. Here are my two graduation pictures. I graduated with honors in both degrees.

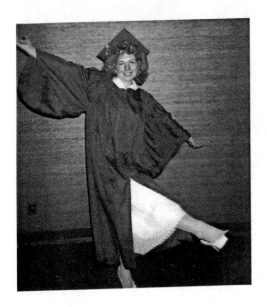

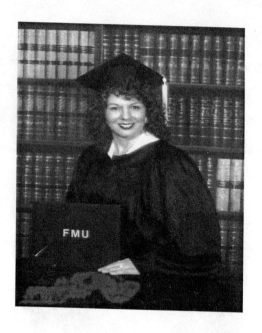

You see my parents, especially my mom, raised me to strive to be *"normal"* and not let my epilepsy be a handicap or a disease. I honor her wisdom for instilling that into me while I was so young ! When I called, she was so shocked by my quitting words. She tried to comfort me and calm me down. Then she suggested I call the Mayo Clinic, and investigate if there were any new medications or techniques out there that I could use to control my seizure activity. I agreed to call them the next day. When I did, they started asking me questions I had **NEVER** been asked before in the 22 years I had dealt with the epilepsy ! They said they would put my information in front of a board of doctors who would review it to see if they wanted to take my case. They then said to call back in a week and they would let me know the decision ! I agreed, then proceeded to have 2 more anxiety attacks over that weekend.

Being part of the process of this review, my current neurologist made me come into his office to have an EEG, hoping to find nothing new ! I had another anxiety attack while in his office and in his uncaring manner, he demanded that I stand up from where I was sitting and shaking. I argued with him for a few minutes, but he still demanded that I stand up. When I finally did, I fell directly to the floor, just like I said I probably would; a surprise to him but no surprise to me. When I got home from the appointment, there was a message on my answering machine from the Mayo Clinic in Scottsdale, Arizona. The message said that *"I had been approved and could I be there by Thursday morning"* – *just 3 days from that moment !* I quickly purchased a ticket and proceeded to fly to the Mayo Clinic in Arizona, and took my brother along for support. We spent a week in Arizona having all kinds of tests done; many that had never been done before. The bonus was that we saw much of the state between appointments from Hoover Dam to Sedona and everything in-between.

The day before we were to return to the clinic to hear the results of the tests, we went to Sedona – a very spiritual place in Arizona. As we sat on those red rocks, I prayed to the Lord:

"Please God give me an answer as to what I am to do. Please help me bring these seizures back under control or help me take them away completely." I then went on to tell God, *"If he/she agreed to make this surgery a*

success, then I would work for the Lord, doing whatever he/she wanted me to do."

Little did I realize the intensity of those words I had said or the depth to which God took them. I tried to wait patiently for an answer (not my strongest feature) and one never came. As we were leaving Sedona, driving back to the hotel, I got my answer – **to *have surgery*** was the only answer God saw at this time in my life. I accepted the answer with much courage and trust, knowing God would never steer me wrong. I was so excited to think I could have a life without any more seizures and I could finally be *"normal,"* (so I thought.)

As we waited patiently for the doctors during my appointment time, I prayed another silent prayer – that my family would be behind me in whatever decision I made. When my neurologist Dr. Hirschorn spoke, she said I had several options, now that my test results were back:

First – I could try traditional drugs.
I said "they won't work, they haven't
in 22 years." *Second* she said, I could try
test drugs. I said "those won't work; they
are drugs in the early stages." A*nd lastly* I
could have surgery. I said, *"there is only
one option– surgery is the answer !"*

She tried to warn me there could be
some side effects; that it might not work;
that the seizures may not go completely
away or they could actually get worse; that
I might regress back to a young age; that I
might not talk, walk or be normal. I
exclaimed without any hesitation in my
voice, *"surgery is the only answer. How
soon can I have it done ?"* I then told her
about my experience with God in Sedona.
She agreed to schedule my surgery for **2
weeks** from that moment. *I was ecstatic !
I could hardly wait for my new life –
seizure free !!* I would finally be living
freely and could actually be *"NORMAL !"*
What an exciting life I would have ! She did
finally encourage me by telling me I would

probably have an *80% chance of being seizure free with this surgical procedure. That percentage was good enough for me !!*

This is the last picture I have of myself, prior to surgery.

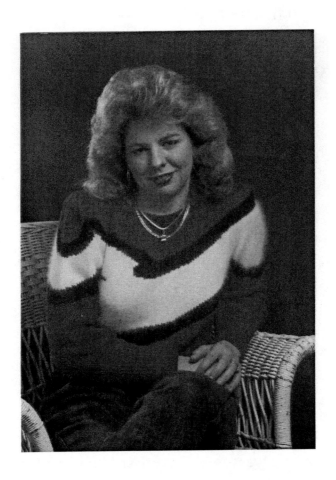

So we went home to get things in order, and I called my parents to tell them my decision. I honesty think they were shocked, surprised, and scared all in the same breath ! I never had a doubt about this procedure, because God told me to do it. *My only fear was that I was going to lose all my hair ! Being a make-up artist, I needed my hair !*

After a week of testing and inducing seizures, the doctors found the area from which my seizures originated. I was fortunate that mine only came from one area, which would make surgery easier, so they said. The last test was when they put a short-term drug in my veins called Phenobarbital, and then they asked me a series of questions to see how I would respond to the drug.

The questions were, "D*o you know where you are ? What is your name ? What is the doctor's name ? Where was I ? and What are we doing ?*" At first I just nodded to all the questions. Then at 42 seconds into the test I began to speak – *"I am at the Mayo Clinic in Scottsdale, Arizona; My name is Susan Lanning; You are Dr. Hirschorn and I JUST PASSED THIS TEST – WE ARE HAVING SURGERY TOMOR - ROW !!"* By speaking within the allotted time, this told the doctors that my speech was on the right side of my brain and not the left, like most people. This would allow them to be more aggressive in my surgery, meaning they could take what they needed until they got it all, since they were not going to hurt my speech.

I was so excited !!

You see the right side of my brain realized at an early age that my left side wasn't doing its job and functioning fully, so it took on all the left sided responsi - bilities. I guess that was one advantage to having seizures so young and early in life !

The morning of the surgery I was so calm and at peace with myself. When the neurosurgeon Dr. Zimmerman came into the pre-op room, he stopped by to see how I was doing and if I needed anything. I said I was fine, but I wanted to see my mom one more time to tell her I was going to be okay. You see I met Dr. Zimmerman the day before, and he told me, not only about the procedure he was going to do, but that *he was only a vehicle for the Lord-that God was the one doing the surgery !...* ***and what a blessing that was to hear !!*** My mom was brought in and I told her I was going to be fine; that God was going to be with us and that this was the right decision ! She smiled quietly and tried to hold her strong presence with me as she had in so many other times in my life.

    The surgery was a success !!!

    After 8 hours of surgery and taking out 3 pieces of my brain, the EEG test went silent – meaning there was **NO MORE** seizure activity in my brain. Upon waking up from surgery, *my only concern was* ***"where was my hair ?"*** I started buzzing the nurses, demanding a mirror. ***"Hair,***

where is my hair ?" was all I could say.
Finally Dr. Zimmerman came in with a
mirror behind his back, saying "did you
request this ?" I said *"yes !! Hair ! Where is
my hair ?"* I repeated. Once I looked in the
mirror I realized my entire head was
bandaged and that was why I didn't feel
my hair. *"OH !!" Was my response thinking
I must be BALD under the bandages !* Dr.
Zimmerman then proceeded to un-
bandage my head, so I could see my hair. I
had almost a whole head of hair. **I was
delightfully shocked, and ever so
thankful !** The piece they shaved was only
seven inches long by two inches wide !
Wondering, I then asked, **"did you get it
all ?"** Dr. Zimmerman, with his quiet smile
and super bedside manner responded with
a simple, *"Yes !!"*

I was overly excited at that point. I
felt so much better, now that I found out I
still had hair and the surgery was a
success. I told him he could bandage me

back up, but he said it was ok to leave it undone.

THE EARLY DAYS OF RECOVERY AND RE-LEARNING CHAPTER 3

My first "hallucination" was in the hospital while I was under 24-hour constant EEG monitoring (brainwave recordings). It occurred because they had reduced my medication intake and were trying to bring on my seizures. By having a seizure while under observation, they could find the spot in my brain, which was triggering the seizure activity. The first one was on Tuesday, October 6th; and it was mainly body jerking for 1½ hours. It stopped after the nurses gave me a shot of Valium. This one was not *"visual,"* just muscle jerking. The first visual hallucin - ation happened two days later on Thurs - day, October 8th, and I felt very scared because I could visually see someone pushing me into an ice hole. The nurses said they talked to me the whole time, but I didn't respond. I was trying to turn over in my bed, as I was trying to climb out of this ice hole that these people kept shoving me into. The people had masks on and when I asked what they wanted, they responded that they hated me and wanted me dead. I didn't understand why, and I asked them to take their masks off. They did and they were people like my brother, my ex-husband and friends I thought I knew and trusted. These people had never hit me or threatened me before, *so why now ?* When the Valium finally took effect and my hallucination stopped, it was 1 hour and 15 minutes later. I was ex - hausted, cold and scared to death. I lay in a tight ball for a long time because I was actually scared for my life. After several more seizures and hallucinations, the doctors found the *"spot"* in my left temporal lobe where the residual seizure activity was coming from.

Yet the surgery was a success !! It just took a little time for the after-shocks to end. I stayed in the hospital about a week and Mom and I played many board games, trying to get my coordination back. After I got discharged from the hospital, Mom and I moved into a nearby hotel for another week, just to make sure every - thing was going to be okay before flying back to California. Thank God my mom was there with me because I needed her love and support.

Now my new life could begin, so I thought ! I could finally be *"normal."* Little did I know how long and hard the recovery was going to be ! Because I regressed mentally and emotionally back to the day before my first seizure, I literally was 2 years old in a 25-year-old body, and boy was life a challenge !!

So there I was...a quarter of a century old, with a 2 year-old brain, living alone, self-employed, trying to figure out life, and recover from surgery all at the same time ! My parents lived in England.... a big 6000 miles away, and my brother was over a 3 hour drive away. I'm sure you would never let your 2-year-old wash your undies, cook your dinner and balance your checking account, but I had to ! Now you can see the challenges I had to deal with !

Little did any of us realize I would have migraine headaches for **16 months, 24 hours a day !!** I finally felt **"real pain,"** for the first time, because when I had epilepsy, I didn't feel any. All of a sudden I didn't have any way to *"check-out,"* when my stress got too high or a situation was out of my control. Now I had to find new tools for me to deal with life, and it was an ongoing challenge ! It took me **6 long years** to catch up mentally and emotion - ally with my chronological age, growing up 6 years for each year following ! Luckily I learned quickly because I was eager; just a one time lesson and deja vous took over ! I went through puberty in 6 months not 6 years like most, which actually was a very nice side benefit ! I moved numerous times over this ten year period, trying to find answers to speed up my healing. I yearned to *"be normal !!"* I still don't know what that means and *ironically, as of today, I have decided I like being DIFFERENT !!*

I returned home after surgery on Thursday October 22nd. I slept on the plane most of the way home and was in pretty good spirits most of the day, until I had a reaction to the salmon I had for dinner and ended up having to go to the emergency room to get a Benadryl shot to stop the reaction. I did quite well the first weekend, except I had a lot of cold sensations and auras, but **no seizures**. An aura is a feeling or a warning one gets before they have a loss of consciousness and laps into a seizure. It had barely been a month since surgery and I was feeling all kinds of new and strange emotions; emotions I had never felt before.

The next hallucination happened on Monday, October 26th, four days after arriving back in California. I had gone into my office to look for something and as I stepped into the walk-in closet I had a "hallucination" that someone was hitting me with a baseball bat. So I jumped out of the closet and stood in the middle of the room. The next thing I remember was lying on the floor crying (I had fainted and I think I hit my head on the chair). Mom heard me and came running in to help me, not knowing what was happening in my mind and thus not understanding the hallucination. She quickly got me into a hot bath to try to calm me down; not knowing the waking nightmare was still going on while I was in the tub. She couldn't grasp the idea of this being so real, because she couldn't see the visual drama going on or anyone physically hurting me. Approximately 45 minutes later, I got out of the bathtub, escaped to the couch, and was just holding myself. I was trying to convince myself, (my adult self) and my inner child that I was going to be all right. Mom held me and hugged me but was beside herself because she had never experienced or witnessed a "hallucination" before. A couple hours later she wanted me to talk to my brother and my ex-husband, because they both were in this hallucination saying *"you don't deserve to live and I want you dead."* She wanted them to reinforce the fact that they were not going to hurt me and they didn't want me dead.

A couple of days later, I spoke to Dr. Hirschorn, my neurologist, and she said the hallucination was *"normal,"* and it was my body's way of reacting to the surgery. After talking to her, I felt much better and proceeded to have a good evening. I assumed the head-trips were going to stop, but they didn't. The next one happened as I was sitting all alone in my family room, just working a jigsaw puzzle. Mom was in Sacramento visiting my brother and my father had returned back to New Jersey for work. All of a sudden I felt so alone and horribly scared - in my mind I knew I was fine, but that empty feeling I had inside would not go away. I sat there quietly most of the day trying to understand why I felt so down and out. The only answer I could come up with was that I was jealous of my mom spending time with my brother. I just wasn't feeling loved or supported as much as I needed to feel at that time.

I knew she was physically tired and emotionally drained, but also knew this was the first of many years of *"trying times" still yet to come.* I wondered, did this tiredness give her the excuse to not hug me and kiss me and give me the reassurance I needed during this new beginning of my life that was filled with many scary days ?

I was really having a hard time understanding this. My mom had always been a touchy, kissy, hands-on kind of mom when I was growing up with epilepsy so I didn't understand the extreme change. *Maybe I was spoiled with all the attention I got as a kid, but I loved the hugs and reassurance I always used to*

get - was it wrong to want them now ? I wanted and needed her now, but if every - time I got scared or started to hallucinate, she backed away, or preached at me or left to go play golf, then she might as well go back home to England. I got so scared so easily then, which was something I never really dealt with when I had epilepsy. Why ? This was one of the many new feelings I was going to have to learn to deal with in my recovery. I never really dealt with many feelings like, fear, anger or loneliness when I had epilepsy. I had epilepsy for so long, I was pretty comfortable with it. Now it was gone and I couldn't depend on it or hide behind it anymore.

I felt so angry. How was I to deal with this feeling ? It was so hot, so sharp and painful inside me. "Please make it go away," I said. "I don't like this feeling at all. Why am I feeling this strange way all of a sudden ? I never felt like this before the surgery."

By now my hallucinations had gone from one here or there, to 1 - 2 every day.

My next one happened on Friday of that same week. I was again working a jigsaw puzzle, when my jigsaw picture turned into a hallucination. I tried to work the puzzle faster to get ahead of it, but that didn't help. Finally I got enough strength to stand up and walk away. When I returned to the puzzle the hallucination was just ending and was writing *"the end"* all over the puzzle. This hallucination was going on while Mom was on the phone with my brother. We were supposed to go up the next day and see him - not realizing at the time that it was going to take 2 ½ hours for me to get ready. I kept seeing him saying *"he hated me and wanted me dead, because I took his parents from him in his younger years due to my epilepsy taking priority over his sports."* (At least that was what I was being told during this hallucination.) I told Mom later about the hallucination and that he needed her for support, friendship and advice, and that he needed her as a friend to love him and hold him. I felt badly because I might have caused these hurt feelings inside him.

I awoke a few days later with a migraine headache; one bad enough for prescription pain pills. After eating breakfast, mom told me we were going back to Sacramento to talk with my brother about these hallucinations, since he was in them. I was not thrilled, because we had been up there a few days ago with the intent of talking and it didn't happen. He was busy getting ready for Halloween at that time and I was fine helping out until they turned on that hard rock n' roll music which gave me an instant headache. I proceeded to go to the car to relax, and listen to softer music which would calm me down. Since living alone, I was not used to being around two young boys and lots of noise.

Mom came out to check on me and I told her I just needed to calm down and rest. A few minutes later she re-appeared, and convinced me to come inside to eat dinner. I agreed and came inside to eat, but ended up dealing with one of the boys kicking me. This kicking brought back very vivid memories of one of my halluci - nations, where I remember the kids being told to kick me, hit me and throw things at me because I deserved it ! After he kicked me once, I told him to stop, but he proceeded to kick me again. I wanted to hurt that boy some way, some how - just because of what it represented to me in that hallucination. Not long after that incident, we left. I was very quiet and fought a lot of inner feelings all the way home. This is why I didn't want to go back up there again. I proceeded to go take a bath and ended up having another hallucination in the bathtub. After it was over, I laid on my bed crying, because I was scared and feeling threatened. I was feeling forced to go back into a bad situation and family environment again, and I didn't want to do it. My brother had twisted what I had said just a couple days prior, stating that I was the only feeling guilty because I didn't think I got enough attention in my childhood and I needed to deal with it. Unfortunately, my mom believed my brother over me and con - tinued to for years to come after that ! I felt very alone; I was feeling like a victim for a situation I was already hurting from.

Mom left the room for a while, then came back to give me a hug, and then left again to go straighten up the family room. She then proceeded to tell me to stop crying, and if I wanted anymore hugs I had to come out into the family room and get them ! I just laid there for a long while and ended up going into another hallucination. This time I was in the middle of nowhere; a desert maybe, with no one and nothing around to help me.

I started to cry realizing I was *ALL ALONE* and *ALL BY MYSELF ! I had to survive by myself.... and that meant from NOW ON !!*

I made a big step the next day; I allowed someone not only to touch my head, but also to cut my hair ! I lost my energy not long after that, (like Samson in the Bible) and became quite irritable, especially with myself ! We went to a craft store where I got easily frustrated with the details involved in cross-stitch, something I used to love to do. Mom and I finally returned home, and I rested before venturing out to give a scarf presentation to a group of business ladies. I did fine on the presentation, but getting ready was a true ordeal ! I couldn't decide what to wear, as my clothes seemed too bold for me now and putting on make-up was something else. It all made me feel like a hooker ! I used to be able to do make-up in 4 minutes in the dark with no problems. This night it took me 24 minutes and I still wasn't sure if I liked it. I hadn't worn make-up since the 3rd of October and had for - gotten how to put it on ! *What a disaster !!*

Moving forward, I had my first *"longest day"* since prior to surgery. I went to the flea market with my mom and best friend. We thought we would only go for a couple of hours, but I lasted longer. I did great until I had an anxiety attack. I walked across the way to look at a booth, leaving my mom and friend on the other side. I was fine until I turned around and I could not see them. I got scared and started to feel my chest tighten like I couldn't breathe. I felt like they had brought me there to drop me off and leave me there. I tried to convince myself that wasn't true and I made myself leave the booth and go find them. As soon as I got outside of the booth, I saw my mom coming towards me; I was fine after that ! We did a couple of other stores and returned home some 8 hours later. I got tired very quickly upon returning home, so I took a hot bath to relax. I told mom of the anxiety attack I had earlier. She was shocked, and didn't even realize that I had had one !

Dad came in from China on Nov 5th, one day before my birthday ! He was in charge of all of Europe and Asia for his company at that time so he traveled most of the time. I had not seen him since July, so he made a special trip to be there for my birthday ! He brought me some jewelry from his travels abroad, and I was so tickled and felt so special ! I didn't do much as my migraines were terrible and very debilitating. Unfortunately, my father had never been sick in his life, so he had no understanding or compassion for people who were ill or in pain. *"Take 2 pills and go back to work,"* was his attitude. Unfortunately, that didn't always work, especially for me !

Then came November 6th, my 25th birthday. I was 3 weeks out of brain surgery and two days shy of a month free of seizures ! My seizures had actually stopped on October 8th, five days before my surgery ! My parents threw me a party, per my request. I wanted the party more so for my friends, so I could say thank all of them for all of their support and prayers while I went through the surgery. I had a good time and got to visit with lots of buddies. I was 25 years old, feeling and acting like a 2-year-old most of the time.... *boy did I not realize how hard this ordeal was going to be !*

I wanted to go back to the Mayo Clinic, to talk to the neurologist or psychiatrist so I could better understand all these feelings inside of me. Mom didn't want to go, but with all of these emotions inside, I just wanted someone to explain them to me. Mom didn't even plan on being around for my open house of my BeautiControl business. I felt hurt. She acted like she was all excited and able to help, but then she backed down, which gave me a false sense of security. "Is it okay to be scared ?" I asked myself. "As soon as I began to feel *"normal"* or like a *"big girl / adult"* I got scared and upset...why ?"

So I prayed, "Please Lord help me get over these feelings. I don't like them !! Please Lord give me the answer to these questions so I can better understand and do a better job in dealing with them.

Dear Lord, why can't I "just deal with it, just handle it, and just let it go ?" It sounds so easy, but how do I actually do it ? I wasn't taught that in my early lifetime, so why should I know it now in this **new lifetime ?"** Dear Lord, help me know it now !!"

Here's another prayer I wrote to God that same day:

"Please Lord, help me feel stronger and not so anxious.
Please give me the strength to grow, the wisdom to know and understand and the patience to learn what I need to.
I know there is a light at the end of the tunnel, but the light gets dim so often, or there's a bend in the road.

*Please give me the love and support and
reassurance I need to continue to grow
stronger and stronger each and every day;
To understand days like today and feelings I
encountered today.
Love me and hold me close - don't let me fall
and stray too far from home or grounds I am
familiar with.* **AMEN"**

So why was I still having these
hallucinations ? I was taking the medi -
cation regularly, as prescribed. On
November 17th I had another horrible
hallucination, which lasted about a half-
hour. I was hallucinating that my mom was
telling me I was a bother, a bitch, a pain in
the ass and a waste of her time; then she
pushed me off a cliff !

So I prayed, *"Help me Lord, I am so
scared and confused !! My Mom hates me !!"*

I was so afraid I tried to call my
doctor at the Mayo Clinic but my phone
line was dead, just like in those horror
movies ! So I ran to the manager's office at
my complex to use the phone and call my

doctor, but unfortunately, she was seeing patients and I had to call back in 30 minutes ! When I returned back to my apartment, my mom questioned me where I went, who I called and why I didn't get her. I tried to explain to her that I was still in the hallucination when I went to the office, so I did not even know she was there. I had snapped out of it by the time I got to the rental office. I went in my bed - room to cry like I did after every halluci - nation, because I was so shook up and scared from it. *It seemed so real !* Mom came into my bedroom, but she didn't say anything and didn't give me a hug or a kiss. Unfortunately this made the hallucination that much more real to me ! Mom finally returned back to England, to take care of dad and let me fend for myself.

I did go back to Mayo Clinic the following week and got my medication reduced; the first of nine trips in a calendar year ! My best friend went with me, as my mother had returned to England for Thanksgiving with my father. After returning from Arizona and seeing my doctors, I began feeling a little better. My medications were *TOO HIGH*, and THEY were causing the hallucinations and dizziness. I spent Thanksgiving with another girlfriend and her family. She was also in the BeautiControl business.

I spent many of my days with my best friend in BeautiControl, as I had not gotten my drivers license back yet. We became each other's shadows for the next few months, as she drove me to many places. We joined our forces together being in the same cosmetic business and helped each other grow. *The doctors finally returned my driver's license to me in February of 1993.*

One day we went shopping, as I wanted to purchase some more tins and baskets for my Christmas open house that weekend. Also, I wanted to buy some wood to make shelves in my storage room, and add some more track lighting to my office, so we had plenty to do. We finally returned home around 9 PM and we ate the home cooked soup I had made earlier. After eating, she left and I took a walk to the mailbox to get the mail.

After picking it up, I noticed my seizure video from the clinic was there, so I came home and watched it. *Boy was it scary! Those seizures were violent!* No wonder I was always tired afterwards. I understand they were more violent than my *"normal"* ones, which made them even more frightening! Scared, I called my mom after watching it and unfortunately, we ended up in a fight over her opinions and interpretations versus mine. I only wanted to share the video experience with her; I didn't want a lecture on what I wasn't doing right – the right way was her way I guess. I was taking prescriptions pills vs. herbs and vitamins; I wasn't exercising like I should; I wasn't cooking balanced meals; I let my body plan my days (good days and bad). Also I was allowing myself to get down, and I let everyone else tell me how to run and live my life, including her. We ended the conversation with her yelling and arguing with me, and me crying and hanging up. She was very cold at the end and sarcasti - cally said, *"I'm sorry I upset you and that you're crying, but I'm going to hang up."* I told her she wasn't sorry or she wouldn't have gotten me so upset and crying to begin with. Then I hung up on her and started to cry even more. The phone rang 5 minutes later and I wouldn't answer it. I let the answering machine pick up, but no message was left.

I asked myself, *"Why do I let or allow her to upset me so easily, so badly and so much ? Why is she always coming at me and worse yet, comparing me to my brother and his situation ?"* I told myself, *"we may be related by blood but that's it !! I don't think, talk, or act like him, so please don't compare me to him. He is an*

alcoholic and an ex-drug addict and I'm
nothing like him or his living situation !!"

Here are the letters I wrote to my parents, trying to explain how I felt. Since I was having no success in talking to them, I thought writing might be a good altern - ative, but it didn't seem to help at all.

December 12, 1992
Dear Dad,

I know you're shocked to receive a letter from me, but I wanted to discuss something with you. First off, I love you a lot and always will. Second, the other evening I got very upset and shook up because I felt like you didn't see or respect me as an adult, but instead as an immature 3 year old child who needed someone by her side all the time. I know I have my moments where I fall down but I'm old enough to pick myself up now. Please learn to trust me and my judgment on things – whether they are about my well-being, health, or responsibilities. I felt like I needed someone to hold my hand every step of the way (just to walk) the other Monday night but I don't. I know that I sometimes make mistakes and sometimes do the wrong thing, but right now I need to learn to do for myself; to be indepen - dent and to gain confidence in my new life and myself.

I appreciate you being there for me and helping me through those trying times (both financially and emotionally). I'm not saying you're wrong, I'm just asking you to look at me from an adult's point of view to an adult instead of an adult to a helpless child's point of view. I got my feelings hurt when you were being sarcastic to me and said to deal with my own feelings and stop calling you "every 5 minutes" for an answer. I was extremely hurt because I had only called you that one time since Saturday night. I know I was previously calling daily but I'm over that phase in my healing. I'm growing up and don't need daily reassurances from you anymore – I'll be fine. (once I say I'm fine then I'll be fine). I'm sorry I seemed to be calling and bugging you a lot but it was just a phase I was going through !!

I'm not criticizing you; I am just sharing with you how I feel and what I want. I may fall and need a hand up but please don't walk for me. I need to declare my individuality and independence from you all, but I'm not declaring a loss of caring or closeness. My independence means that I can clearly define myself on emotionally important issues, but that doesn't mean emotional distance between us. I want to leave the fighting, instructing, criticizing and adult-to-child like games in our past and start building a sharing, loving, trusting and adult-to-adult relationship for our future. By doing this I can let go of the anger and guilt I hold within me and start the healing process towards a happier and healthier Susan.

I felt guilty writing you this letter because you've done a lot for me (financially and emotionally) and I don't want to hurt your feelings or sound unappreciative because I am, but now its time to let me grow and become the young lady I'm meant to be. Thanks for your support and love. I love you forever !

Love Ya,

Susan

December 13, 1992

Dear Mom,

I'm writing this letter to clear up some misunderstandings between us. I appreciate your concern and I know its important to you to know I'm well cared for, but I'm struggling hard to learn to be an independent person from both you and dad and from epilepsy. It's important to me to do what I think is best, and I know I'm going to make mistakes and bad choices – but I need to do it to learn for the next time. I want your support in allowing me to do that and also to allow me to express my feelings and opinions. I can't grow and mature if you don't allow me to express my feelings without thinking I'm always "lashing out" at you.

I still need your support both emotionally and financially, but I'm getting stronger and better every day. I don't want to fight, contradict, or be at wits end with you. I'm learning not only to listen but to express myself better too. I know you're older and

65

wiser than I am, but I'll get there. I need your support to help me adjust to my new life and get me through these trying times.

Please don't criticize or condemn me for wanting to express my feelings. I don't want to hurt you ever, but I'm hurt inside and I'm scared. Everything is very new and very different to me and it's taking some time (and lots of patience) to adjust to. I'm trying to rebuild my confidence and security from within and some days I need more reassurance and love than others.

I'm not criticizing you; I'm just sharing with you how I feel and what I want. I want you to treat me like an adult, not an immature 3 year old. I know I have my moments where I fall but please only offer your hand – don't walk for me. I appreciate you being there to help me through these trying times (both emotionally and financially). I need to declare my individuality and independence from you all, but I'm not declaring a lack of caring or closeness. Please just stand beside me and be my friend and supporter – don't stand in front of me and be the leader or behind me and be the follower.

I'm not writing this to hurt you – I just need a moment of your time to listen to me as an adult who is trying to express her feelings in the best way she knows how. I love you and I always will.

Love Ya,

Susan

Another typical rough day, I woke up with a migraine again and I could only stay up 2 hours before returning to bed for 2 more hours. Upon waking, I got up and got my shower because I had an open house that day from 4 PM to 9 PM at the clubhouse. Unfortunately, no one came, so I read my book and closed up around 7:45 PM vs. 9:00 PM. It was probably a blessing in disguise, because I still didn't feel good. So I spent the rest of the night easy. I had a message from my doctor in Scottsdale and she sounded upset with me. That shook me up a bit so I called another gal who had surgery about the same time I did and we talked about it. I finally survived the day. Later on I had another open house and sold 10 baskets, which made me $165 in sales !

The next day started out fair but then I got a headache. I took the new pill and it seemed to work for a while, but just as I was closing up, I could feel it coming back. So I took more herbs and another pill. I called my best friend in South Carolina; only to find out she had birthed her baby – a baby boy with lots of hair ! I was so excited to be an *"aunt"* again. After that I went out with my girlfriend for a while and we saw Christmas Tree Lane in Ceres, a small town nearby, which was really neat.

Upon coming home I started to get my headache again, so I called mom and then went to bed. Unfortunately, my conversation with Dr. Hirschorn who I finally spoke to, was still on my mind. I dozed for a couple hours, but couldn't

sleep much. By then it was 4 AM and un -
fortunately I was wide awake, so I wrote
this letter apologizing for all of my phone
calls and extra stress I was causing them.
Then I tried to sleep again.

Here is the letter I wrote to my
doctors, apologizing for bothering them
so much.

December 18, 1992

*Dear Dr. Hirschorn, Dr., Zimmerman and the
Neurology Dept.*

*I wanted to take this time to say thanks
and I'm sorry. A thanks is for all the support
you've given me over these last 2 months. A
thanks is for performing the surgery and
giving me a chance to live a* **"normal"** *life. A
thanks is for all your patience in answering all
my questions and addressing all my fears and
doubts. I know I go through phases where I call
a lot and I'm sorry – I just get scared because
everything is so new to me. All the pains,
feelings and fears are all new and sometimes
overwhelming.*

I'm doing my best to deal with everything but sometimes I just need extra support or an answer to why I'm feeling the way I am. I am sorry for the after-hour calls. Unfortunately new pains or fears develop and I don't know what to do or how to deal with them. I live alone so I don't have someone with me at all times to help me deal with all of these new changes. I know deep down I'll be okay but sometimes I just get scared and don't know what to do, so unfortunately, I call you all for advice or guidance. I'm hoping that this was only a phase and one that I've grown out of by now.

Please bear with me and understand where I'm coming from. I'll try to deal with the situations better in the future and on my own without bugging you all the time. I just have never met such loving and caring doctors as you all and unfortunately I became attached to your caring nature very quickly.

I'm trying to stand on my own two feet but I fall sometimes – some days more than others. I apologize for all the phone calls during the day and the late at night too. I'm getting stronger every day; some days are

*tougher and scarier than others are, but I'm
going to make it.*

*I just want to say thanks for being
patient with me. I'm going to be okay now.
Thanks for taking the time to answer my
questions and to help me get rid of the
migraines - or at least be able to control them.*

*I feel so lucky to be given this chance to
live life without seizures. Thanks for changing
my life. My future looks brighter and it's
coming soon. Thanks again for everything.*

Susan Lanning

It was a few days till Christmas and
my parents had just arrived from England
around 7:30 PM They both looked tired, so
dad was in bed by 9 PM (5 AM their time)
and mom followed around 10:30 PM. The
next morning, they were both up by 6:30
AM; I woke up at 8 AM. We went to break -
fast and then shopping at the Mall, the
jewelry store and Wal-Mart. Then we came
home and I prepped for the BeautiControl
meeting / party. *Wow, I thought, "What a*

day ! It's 11 o'clock and I've got to be up at 6 AM and I'm not even tired ! Maybe I'll wrap gifts."

Three days till Christmas and I was up early to go to a chamber meeting with my best friend. I was trying so hard to build this cosmetic business. After attending our meeting, we ran several errands before returning home. I took a 20 minute power nap when I got home, to get some new energy, as I was throwing a surprise party for my parents that night ! I think my parents knew of the party, but they didn't know who was coming.

They were shocked and pleasantly surprised to see all the people I had invited for them. The party was a big success, except I started to get a migraine headache and felt extremely tired. I finished cleaning up the clubhouse and then, following the protocol of what was politically correct, joined the remaining guests in a social chat.

After they left, I returned home, feeling anxious, and went quickly to bed. Mom came and lay beside me, trying to calm me down by giving me advice. The advice wasn't helping the headache at all. I decided I was going for walk, so she returned to bed with dad. While walking, my eyes started to tear and they haven't stopped since then. (Maybe it's my fears being released through the tears.)

As I walked, I reflected *"I feel so alone again...why? Have I grown up and mom can't relate to me as a grown-up? I have tried to explain to her how I feel, but she keeps telling me to do deep breathing and to stop crying. But I want to cry!! I think that is why my eyes are still tearing...I must need to cry!"*

I CRIED OUT, "I JUST WANT A HUG PLEASE!! NO ADVICE, JUST A HUG!!"

I asked God, *"Why am I getting depressed again? I don't like this place, please make it stop!"*

'Twas Christmas Eve and I had to go full blast per my parent's request. Dad wanted me to go grocery shopping with him, and upon returning mom wanted me to go shopping with her too. Unfortun - ately, I fought migraines all day, so I was pretty quiet. She got upset with me, because I used a cuss word. She told me I reminded her of my sister-in-law. That really hurt my feelings. I just shut up after that. I wanted to start crying right there in the mall, but I didn't. Mom seemed to have zero patience with me at that time and yet they wanted me to go to England for a MONTH !!

I told God, "Dear God help me ! I don't mean to sound sarcastic or mean, but when I miss a few words or use a childlike phrase, that's how she reacts to it...sarcastically. Why is my relationship with her falling further and further by the wayside ? Is it becoming more and more distant ? Doesn't she love me anymore ? I'm trying so hard to get well and grow up. Can't she see that ?"

Here is the prayer I wrote to God:

"Dear God, please help me to retain my love and friendship I used to have with my mother. PLEASE !!!"

Merry Christmas to you too !!

Unfortunately, I woke up to a terrible migraine headache. My father, a morning person, asked me how I was as soon as I got out of bed. I said, *"I'm ok."* He quickly commented back, *"what does that mean ?"* It was like he didn't comprehend that I was not a bright-eyed morning person, never have been, probably never will be, so I wasn't sure how I felt yet ! He was so used to just hearing *"I'm fine...having a great day"* and then giving a political smile back, but that's phony, isn't it ? I just wasn't sure if I was *"fine"* yet.

Santa was good to all of us, but my migraine kept me under the weather, allowing no real enthusiasm for anything. I spent the rest of the afternoon and eve - ning with my ex-husband, as I was not in any shape to travel 2 hours to Sacramento for a social party. I enjoyed his company and friendship. He had become a better friend to me going through this surgery, then he was the whole time we were married, which wasn't a long time.

My parents were in and out of my house for the next five days like social butterflies; I hardly saw them. They had golf games and social parties to attend to. *I was so glad to spend so much time with them while they were there, **sarcastically speaking !*** Mom made a comment that she didn't think I wanted to be around them or spend time with them. She was ***SO WRONG !*** I had only asked them to stay in Sacramento for the first two days, so I could plan their surprise Christmas party that I threw for them ! So I told myself, "I think I will just shut up. I seem to cause too many unintentional problems by talking or trying to explain myself and my actions."

Here are two prayers I wrote and said to God:

"Dear God, I feel so alone and I feel like I am being made out to be a mean person who is white trash and enjoys hurting people. I didn't think I was that way, but Lord If I am...

PLEASE help me change because I wouldn't hurt a fly on purpose, let alone a person !"

"Dear God, why doesn't my mom understand me ? Why can't she see I am hurting deep inside and I just want her to hug me and kiss me and make it all better like she used to do when I was a little girl. Why does she run away from me when I am scared, instead of coming closer and embracing and comforting me ? Have I lost my mom forever ? Did this surgery make my mom walk away from me forever ? **PLEASE LORD, ANSWER ME !"**

I was to head back to the Mayo Clinic in Arizona the next week for a check-up on my migraines. They thought I might have a leak in my brain. My best friend offered to go with me, and I felt I might take her up on the offer, as my mom and I were still fighting and I was not sure I could deal with a constant battle in Arizona. I definitely did not want to go to England and be stuck there, fighting and bickering all the time...in a foreign country far away from home ! I hoped the doctors would find a leak. At least then we would have a reason for these migraines and I could be done with them.

They found a small nasal drip and gave me medication for it, and they reduced my anti-seizure medications, as they were too high once again ! *YEA !* Unfortunately, my migraines continued for *16 SOLID MONTHS*, much of the time without any relief. Eventually, I was off *ALL of my anti-seizure medication 9 months after surgery ! At least that part was a blessing !*

I spent New Year's Eve with my ex-husband. We watched a movie and played some card games after I made cheese enchiladas. Then he sang to me all night long...watch out heart...that's how he hooked me the first time ! We reminisced over old times, the last ten years and how we had changed and where our lives had gone. We had become better friends, more so then we ever were in our dating and married years.

We took dad to the airport on the second of January and mom stayed on for a couple more weeks. I prayed we wouldn't fight and bicker the whole time, because I couldn't take that kind of stress ! We did pretty well; had our moments both good and bad, but she finally left, and it was quiet again...a sound I was learning to love !

I attended our BeautiControl Regional Convention in Los Angeles for a few days in late January. I was so excited, energized, and ready to work again - thank God ! I won a double inventory order while there, so that set my sails and me flying ! Upon returning from the convention, I called my doctor and asked to get my driver's license back, as not having it was causing me a lot of stress and I couldn't really work my business properly without it. She said she would discuss it with the other doctors.

I was admitted back into the hospital in Arizona in mid-February 1993. I was still having migraine headaches 24 hours a day; major mood swings; and in addition was now having fainting spells. They wanted to make sure I wasn't having seizures that were masking themselves as fainting spells. *I was not, just fainting spells !!* I was under 24-hour constant camera observation, as they were hoping to catch these anxiety attacks on tape. Unfortunately, I was now going on almost 4 months of constant migraines, depres - sion and little or no sleep, rendering me frustrated and worn out !

I was upset and had no energy. I thought the surgery was going to give me a new life, not a worse one ! Around 10:30 PM, I got really mad, more frustrated and was having major feelings of despair so I swallowed 6 pain pills, instead of 2 ! I had been hiding them in my drawer all day, in case I decided to commit suicide ! I was at my wits end and did not care anymore ! It

had been 4 horrendous months of my life.
Between the anxiety attacks, migraines 24
hours a day, hallucinations, depression
and now the fainting spells – **I was fed**
up *!! I had already told the doctor I wanted*
my seizures back. At least I knew how to
deal with them and live life accordingly !

After taking the 6 pills, my heart
started to race, and then I went through a
terrible anxiety attack. The anxiety attack
was so bad they had to restrain me and tie
me down, and administer Valium through
my veins. It lasted for a couple of hours.
All of this was being recorded on tape.
After the anxiety attack finally ended I
dozed off for a while, but the headache
only eased - it never went away !

Dr. Hirschorn, my neurologist, was
extremely upset with me the next morning
when she learned of what I tried to do, as
seen on camera. I tried to explain my side,
but she didn't want to hear it. She was just
telling me how frustrated she was with me
and my recovery because of the constant

phone calls and now a suicide attempt, in the hospital !

After this suicidal attempt, Dr. Nelson, the psychiatrist, who had been treating me so far, wanted me admitted to the psychiatric ward at the Mayo Clinic in Rochester, Minnesota. He wanted me to spend a month there, learning new tools and skills to re-adjust to my new life with - out seizures. I was willing to give it a try, but my insurance would not cover it and my parents were not game to foot the bill. The psychiatrist put me on an anti-depres - sant called Elavil that finally helped me sleep, a lot ! I stayed in the hotel for a few days after checking out of the hospital, hoping to get approved to go to the Mayo Clinic in Minnesota, which never happened.

Finally, I returned to California and was told to check-out the psychiatric center in my town. It would probably do the job; just not have Mayo doctors running it. I definitely needed some help adjusting to this new identity and life without seizures. So on February 25th, I went to check out this psychiatric center and see what they had to offer. *While I was investigating them, they checked me in !!* Since I still had suicide thoughts, they admitted me immediately and made me a Q15 status, which means I was to be checked on every 15 minutes ! The first day was pretty easy, but it was all down hill after that !

We did many group sessions and had to explain why we were there and why we needed help. In one of my groups, which my caseworker ran, we talked about our losses in this lifetime. I talked about my surgery, my divorce and the adjust - ment to life without seizures. She quickly reminded me about the loss of family support, as my family had moved to England. We also spoke of me playing *"the china doll,"* and *"the puppet with strings"* and how I tried to please others and do what was expected of me, which was not always what I wanted to say or do. This was the first of many attempts to break through to me, and to try to tear down the mask I was so accustomed to hiding behind !

Mom was back in the states and she came up after dinner to see me. We started to talk, but she got defensive and so I shut down on her. I tried to explain to her we all have different problems, some more than others do, but we can all still listen to each other and share with each other. *She just felt like I was hanging the family out to dry for the entire world to see...like we had some major family secret that I wasn't supposed to talk about !*

I fainted and had another anxiety attack on that Friday night. This attack lasted 2 1/2 hours ! I got very little sleep and woke up dizzy and with a headache. After returning to bed and taking some medications, I got up and attended a group session. This counselor knew how to push people's buttons and she was doing a great job with mine ! My legs shook a lot and I had a continuos smile on my face. The counselor saw this and tried to break through. She said I needed to let the mask down and see who the lady inside was, but I was scared ! There were so many un-familiar feelings inside me, that I didn't know if I wanted to meet her ! After that group session I was still shaking and dizzy, so I decided to go lie down. I fainted on my way to my room and then proceeded to have another anxiety attack.

The nurse held me for a long time, while I was having the attack; it felt very comforting and secure ! She said she knew what caused these anxiety attacks. I asked what, but at first she wouldn't answer me. She later came back into my room and told me she thought my subconscious brought them on to get attention, much like my seizures used to get me. At first, I denied her thoughts, as I would never consciously bring on a seizure or anxiety attack. I thought about it long and hard and dis -

cussed it with many people that evening. I decided she was right. I didn't do it consciously, but unconsciously I could see it. So I decided I was going to work on being my own best friend and looking within or to God for the answers.

I stayed eight days and I learned a lot about myself and made many new friends. *I started to crack away at this con -stant smiling mask I had worn for over 24 years.* The lady underneath was almost a stranger to me. She had many built-up feelings from the past that I never even knew existed. **She was so angry, scared, and confused – I wasn't sure I wanted to get to know her !**

Here you can see how I was feeling, as I started to *"take my mask off."* **This was tough, exhausting, and very scary to me !**

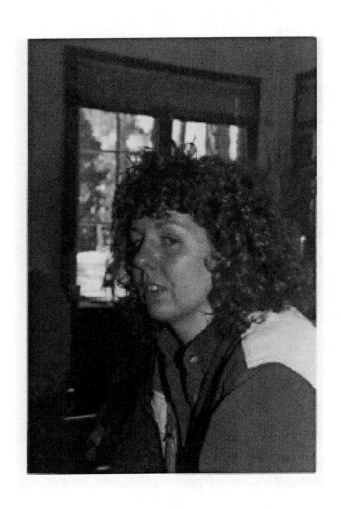

THE FEELINGS OF ANGER, FEAR AND DESPAIR, FEELINGS I HAD NEVER FELT BEFORE - CHAPTER 4

After leaving the psychiatric center in late February 1993, I got my license back and my parents bought me a red 1992 Geo Storm– it was beautiful and sporty ! *YEA !!* I started attending out - patient therapy on a weekly basis, as it was tough adjusting to being alone after being around people all the time. I dis - covered I was definitely a *people person* !! I made a few good friends while there, some I could really relate to.

In April, the psychiatrist officially diagnosed me with *bi-polar depression*, which really scared me. I tried Zoloft, an anti-depressant drug, but after hearing the doctor's full prognosis, I got really scared and called my parents. They were travel-ling in Hong Kong at the time and I told them I wanted to come home to live with them in England in hopes of beating this.

The flight over there was 18 hours long and I was exhausted, had a migraine and was super scared ! I stayed for three weeks, fought major mood swings while there, and it didn't get any easier at all ! The weather was cold, wet, and dreary all the time, not good for either my migraines or my moods. I was also having crying spells, and suicide attempts, which frightened and frustrated my parents totally !

I returned back to the states at the end of May and enrolled in college for summer school. *Boy was I going against the odds – out of brain surgery for only 7 months, out of school for 4 ½ years, and fighting depression on a daily basis !* Neither the doctors nor I knew how I would do in school. *Well I did wonderfully ! I took two summer school classes in college, drove 100 miles roundtrip 5 days a week, and pulled a 3.4 GPA !* I didn't take *"easy"* classes either. I took Business Law and Microeconomics ! Everyone was amazed, including me ! I had never felt so alive and happy in all of my recovery time as I did in that month of June ! I even went back to Arizona for an 8-month check-up between midterms and finals and my results were outstanding ! *I had actually increased my IQ a few points and my coordination was super.*

Unfortunately, that all came to a screeching halt on July 4th ! I had to spend that holiday alone and I didn't realize how badly it would affect me. The next week I found out I had blood in my other breast, similar to what I had the year before. So I decided to go see my best friend in South Carolina, prior to having surgery, hoping to lighten up and have a good time. Fortunately or unfortunately, we had too good of a time, and when I returned home on Tuesday, I was totally depressed again by Wednesday night, with breast surgery scheduled for Thursday !

I had to drive myself to the hospital - I was really scared and depressed ! Hardly anyone called to check on me. I was in a lot of pain, scared and suffering with depressions and migraines...*ugh !!* I finally recovered and decided I was going to attend the BeautiControl Conference in Dallas, Texas. I felt like I needed some new motivation and techniques to jump-start my business again.

I continued to struggle with my new identity and life I was trying to re-create. This picture was taken in August 1993 at the BeautiControl Convention in Dallas, Texas. *I was 10 months out of surgery at this time. **See how short my hair was !***

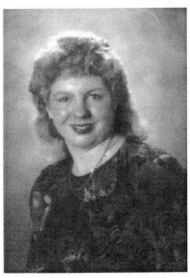

I wanted to move back to the Carolinas, hoping to relive that wonderful week with my best friend from college and her kids and maybe to learn to live a little slower paced life and really start to heal too ! But my parents didn't like the idea, so I returned back to college that fall. Thinking I was *"super student,"* I took 5 full time classes, tried to do an internship at the zoo, and keep my cosmetic business going too. Much to my surprise, I was not ***"super student !"*** To help, I decided to move closer to the campus in Stockton California, because the fog in the winter was horrible and I didn't want to be driv - ing in it.

Unfortunately, I was exhausted and overwhelmed with migraines and depres - sion. So I never got completely organized or unpacked. I kept fighting these daily suicide thoughts and tendencies through - out the entire fall season, and my grades reflected it. *I was flunking almost every -*

thing I touched, quite different from the
summer session !

   Going through all these changes,
challenges, and adjustments I was really
very scared and overwhelmed; yet I didn't
really know how to ask for help properly.
So I would do dumb things to get attention
such as: drink lots of alcohol, (which I had
never done in my epileptic years,) and try
to commit suicide, with an over-dose of
pills. I did this just to get attention and to
feel loved, but it never worked. I remem -
bered it worked for my brother, so I
thought I would try it !

   Just shy of my 1year anniversary in
October 1993, I dropped out of school and
decided to move back to the Carolinas to
be near my best friend. My mom flew in to
help me pack and move, but unfortunately
my mood swings were too much for both
of us to deal with. I snapped at her a lot,
even though I didn't really mean it ! I just
didn't know how to deal with all of the
feelings and stresses, so I just yelled a

lot !! There were so many feelings bottled up inside of me, and I didn't know how to get them out or how to handle them.

Mom tried her best to help me, but unfortunately, she was ill equipped to do the job properly. Before I moved to the Carolinas, she took me to see an ordained minister who claimed to be a healer. Upon meeting this lady, I was very skeptical and very much a non-believer at the time. She proceeded to give me a healing and said my migraines would ease a little every day, and I would take less and less medication and that they would be *totally gone on the 13th day*. I wanted to believe her, but I was hesitant. Guess we would find out soon enough ! I thanked her and left, knowing we had a 2-hour drive back home. *My migraines did ease up a little every day and on the 13th day, they were gone...just like she told me they would be.* **I was truly amazed and totally ecstatic !**

Since I was moving in early November of that year, it was considered my birthday present by my parents, so I got no cards or gifts. Oh well, I was in the south now and near my best friend ! My best friend made me dinner for my birth - day, so that was cool. When my mom had helped me move out, she and I were getting on each other's nerves. She just didn't understand me at that time, and the pain I was constantly in. She didn't know what to say or do to help me, which I know made her feel helpless at times.

Unfortunately, she decided to return to England, a few days earlier than was originally scheduled, which really hurt me deeply. I felt she was like a mother who runs away from her children when they are in a crisis ! Well, the morning my mother was due to leave, I was in my bedroom trying to figure out how to slash my wrist with a steak knife. When my best friend showed up to take her to the airport, I handed her a 5-page suicide note and Living Will in an envelope, and told her to give it to my mom and have her read it *one day*. Reluctantly, she took it, asking me if I wanted to go with her to take my mom to the airport I replied sharply...."*NO !!*"

When they closed the door, I locked it behind them and then proceeded to take **5 HANDFULS** of hydro-codeine and swallow them, knowing they would make my heart stop and kill me. Well, just as they started to work and force my heart to really speed up before coming to a crash - ing halt, my best friend came running through the patio door – the one door I didn't lock. She proceeded to try to shake me conscious, but I was already zoning out of my body. Most of these details were pretty blurry, except I remember telling her to just let me die as she was calling 911.

I was rushed to the hospital and they pumped my stomach full of liquid char - coal, which makes you get sick to get rid of the drugs in your system. I hallucinated and had anxiety attacks for almost 8 hours in the emergency room, trying to beat myself against the restraining bars of the bed. I was trying to get away from the figures in my hallucinations, and in my writhing, pulled the tube out of my arm three different times. I do remember the doctor coming into my room in the middle of this and asking me what I wanted to accomplish. I told him *"I wanted to kill myself."* He said *"you didn't succeed, now how do you feel ?"* I replied *"shitty !!"* He then left me alone. He later came back, after I had been there for almost 7 ½ hours, and asked me again, and I said *"shitty, but for a different reason."* I had just had a chat with God and had decided maybe I did want to live; *maybe I did have a purpose on this planet after all !* My mom was finally allowed to see me; she looked into the room like she had seen a ghost and I probably looked worse than that ! I was finally released, but had that *"drugged up"* feeling for days !

My mom left to go back to England on her regularly scheduled flight. After she left, I was admitted into an out-patient therapy program that met from 9 AM – 12 PM daily. I was starting to get better, but I was black and blue from my nose to my toes, from all of the thrashing and kicking I did at the hospital. I started to get a little more stable and my migraines finally went away, just like the ordained healing reverend said. **She said they would be gone in 13 days and I tried to kill myself on the 11th day !**

I spent Thanksgiving with my best friend and her family, which was wonder – ful ! I then spent most of my time Christ - mas shopping for seven people – as my mom had given me her shopping list for my brother and his family, since they lived overseas making present buying more difficult. It was way too much work and I ended up getting the flu and laryngitis, but I finished the night before I left to go to England for Christmas ! I stayed up all night packing, so I slept most of the way on the plane.

I was fine until a few hours after landing when my migraines returned ! *"Oh NO !" I cried... "I didn't bring my medication with me !" I thought they were gone forever, but my head was splitting open again ! I thought, "Now what ?"* I wanted to return home right then and there, before Christmas, if we couldn't get the migraines to stop so I could feel a little better. The brisk, cold air in England just aggravated my condition. My mom thought she was the cause of them. I tried to explain to her that she wasn't, but she didn't believe me.

I agonized with the thoughts, "Why can't I be that *"perfect normal daughter,"* that they expect me to be ? ... The *"bubbly daughter"* they have always known ?.... *The one who wears a mask to cover her true feelings and just smiles all the time ?"* Even my father said I was *"no fun"* to be around anymore as I got very quiet when I didn't feel good or had a migraine. Mom always thought I was mad so I tried to explain to her that when I talked she would tell me I was snapping at her and bitchy. So to protect myself, I tried to stay quiet and not hurt anyone's feelings. I couldn't win if I wanted to so I chose silence because the mental and emotional punishment was less !

Then my brother and his family arrived and all the attention went to the kids, totally ! I had done all the shopping for these people and was left wrapping the gifts by myself for over 4 hours. The kids got all the attention, which I tried to understand, but couldn't. *Remember I was emotionally growing at a rate of 5-6 age years per annual year. So I was only 8 years old in emotional years at this time !* I just wanted to be acknowledged for being a human with feelings; was that so wrong ? Why couldn't they just include me in the attention with everyone else ?

We went to a British Christmas party on the 18th, as we were going to celebrate Christmas on the 19th, to accommodate

my brother's family and their needs. The
party was fun, and pleasantly different,
and I got to wear a pretty velvet skirt with
a white silk blouse and black sequined
jacket – something I really enjoyed during
the Christmas holiday. I was going to wear
it on stage at my BeautiControl conference
in January, as I was due to receive 3
awards for promotions I had earned in my
cosmetic company ! We had Christmas the
next night and my parents surprised me
by giving me a gorgeous red leather coat,
which I had seen, in a store window in
South Carolina. That turned out to be the
best part of Christmas...the rest went
down hill quickly !

I just didn't feel like I belonged with
this group. The children tore through their
gifts in 1.5 seconds and then moaned that
they didn't get any more toys. (They had
already opened them on day one of their
arrival.) I couldn't believe my brother
tolerated their actions, but he seemed to

look to our parents to discipline and entertain them.

We went into London to see the Madame Tussad's Wax Museum, which is quite a large tourist attraction. Mom did her thing and hung close to the kids and my brother. My father I saw only occasion - ally and by the time we reached the half - way point to get a drink, they had all dis - appeared. I was trying to stay calm, but deep inside I was getting scared. I felt all alone, maybe lost in a big city, in a foreign country! I then passed my mom and sister-in-law coming from the bathroom. I thought they saw me, but they didn't so they walked right on by me. I couldn't believe my mom was acting so cozy with my sister-in-law after she had physically attacked my mom just less than a year ago. I personally didn't like her, and even more so after she scuffled with my mom and literally pushed her into the fireplace.

As I was standing in the bathroom talking to a lady who had lived in the USA, my sister-in-law abruptly showed up and proceeded to rudely interrupt us. She told me they were waiting for me downstairs, as the kids wanted to eat and they hadn't been able find me. I was stunned and embarrassed, and by the time my sister-in-law left, so was the nice lady. I finished up, went out and didn't see any of them for a few more minutes. Then my father appeared saying that he couldn't find me either, and no one knew where I had gone, and that the least I could do was tell him where I was!

Deep inside I was upset and beside myself, saying "stop yelling at me - stop being so mad at me and treating me so horribly !"

Later, when we went on the ride that takes you into the planetarium, I was quiet like a church mouse. I had a horrible migraine headache, was recovering from the anxiety attack I had in the bathroom just before they showed up, and was feeling quite unloved and "different" around these *"people"* who were supposed to be *my family* ! I couldn't stand it any - more.... so when we left the planetarium, I asked for the house key. My mom told me she didn't have it, so I said I would be home later as I was not going to be treated like a piece of sh** by them, and of all people, my sister-in-law did not have the right to yell at me! My mom *"the peace maker"* in our family, tried to convince me to hang with them...but I said *"no way !"*

I went to Piccadilly Circus, ate lunch, went to the Guinness Book of Records and just walked around looking at shops. I finally got home around 7:30 PM that evening and went straight upstairs to my room without conversing with anyone. When I finally came downstairs, I got the third degree – *"where have you been, what did you do, why did you go by yourself, why didn't you call"*.... etc, etc...I finally cried out *"Just leave me alone !! I don't belong in this crowd !"*

Phew ! That year finally came to an end and I got to return back to the states ! I was so glad to see the south and the nice people again and proclaimed I was never going back to England again !

Thank goodness it was another New Year – 1994 and time to get ready to go to my cosmetic company's conferences. I was going to both the one in North Carolina and the one in California, since I had team players in both areas! I would be getting honored on stage for placing in the *"recruiting promotion"* the company had run that fall. *I placed second in California and third in the Carolinas.* It was great to see all my friends again in California, as we talked a good bit on the phone, but I had missed seeing them in person.

This was a tough year for me. Although I was closer in proximity to my family, they still were a long ways away, as they lived on another continent! I tried hard to figure out what life was all about. I became active in a singles group at the

Baptist church in town; which seemed to help a little bit. I still felt very separated and different, even around these wonder - ful Christian singles. Most of them had never moved out of that town, let alone traveled in America. They were so content with their simple lives, their friends, their time at church and their hourly jobs. Unfortunately, I didn't know what *"being content"* was all about. (Little did I know I would spend the next 6 years finding out and searching the world over for it !) I had already moved 20+ times at the age of 26 ! I wanted more out of my life - so I thought.

During this year in the South, I became a strong believer in Jesus Christ and God, our Father. This was a good thing, considering many times I thought he/she had walked away from me and left me alone. *I was so wrong !* It was during those times of trial and struggle that God was there the most, carrying me, holding my hand, and comforting me to keep moving forward. A new dawn was ahead,

or so I was told in many of my prayer
conversations, but **I lacked patience, big
time! I wanted it NOW !!** I realized that
God had a plan for me, like he does for all
of us down here on this planet called
Earth. I just wished he had filled me in on
the details of those plans, or at least have
given me a sneak peak at what was coming
up !

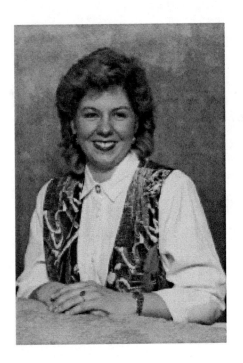

I continued to build my cosmetic and image consulting business, in between my bi-polar swings and moments of des - pair and depression. I stayed in constant contact with my team players in California, through monthly newsletters, bulletins, certificates and prizes for reaching their goals! I really got to enjoy the company of my best friend from college and her two children. I called them *"our children,"* because she got to raise them and I got to be their *"Aunt"* and spoil them ! *As much fun as they were to be around, I quickly realized I was in no way ready to have any of my own at that time. I still needed to finish healing and re-raising myself ! **That was a full-time job in itself !***

I went to Ohio over Easter that year to see the Ordained healing minister and her family. I had grown quite close to her, as she really healed me and helped me turn my life around. I met her daughter and we instantly became friends. I attend - ed church with them on that Sunday and got to listen to *"Mama"* preach. *Boy was she powerful!* I wished a silent prayer that day; I wanted to be just like her. She really seemed to know how to impact the people in the congregation and revive their faith in Jesus. What really made that Easter special was that she was able to give a healing to a little boy, who had been wearing braces on his arms since birth. He asked her to heal him, so he could run like the other kids. She and God healed him that day and he ran happily out of the church as soon as he could. I just sat there and cried. I had witnessed a miracle in front of my own eyes! I knew for sure then that God is good and that God does heal his/her people when we ask as an innocent child because I witnessed it!

This was my turning point in being a full time Christian and believer in our Lord Jesus Christ. I became a devout Christian from that weekend on with a major new dedication in my life!

Here is a picture from that year's BeautiControl Conference.

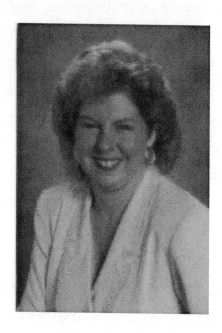

My parents returned from England in October 1994 and moved to New Jersey, back where my dad's corporate head - quarters was located. Mom convinced me to move home; telling me life would be good if she were near me, helping me recover. She could fix my meals, do my laundry, and even help me re-build my cosmetic business in another state. *It*

sounded too good to be true and after moving there I realized it was !

Because she was busy, unpacking and organizing her house, getting ready for the holidays and such, she just didn't have the time and patience with me like I so hoped she would ! Dad worked extremely long hours, like he always did – *"work hard, play hard"* was his motto. He worked 12-16 hour days and then come home on the weekends to play in golf tournaments and entertain friends. So I didn't see much of either of them, and I didn't like the feeling of having a curfew or explaining where I was all the time (*excuse me I was 28 not 12* !) I never had a curfew in my teen years *so why now ?* I couldn't stand it, so I ran away from home many times, not telling anyone where I was going or when I'd be back. I needed my space, my peace and my solitude that I was used to it. That old cliche of **"you can't move back home after you move out"** *is SO VERY, VERY TRUE !!*

As 1994 came to an end, I was making plans to either kill myself or move the heck out of there, quickly ! I spoke to a few friends in California, and decided I was ready to go back; to head for the West Coast and be closer to friends my own age !

In 1995 I was at the 2-½ year mark in my recovery – when I decided to return to California, *"the land of liberalism and new ideas,"* so I thought. I needed to find some answers on how to get well and I only wanted to do it naturally. California is known for being pretty radical and inno - vative at times, and for my situation, that was a good thing. I was depressed, frus - trated and very, very angry and I needed lots of answers and many prayers !

After stopping in New Jersey for only 8 weeks during the winter months, I realized I didn't like the cold weather, or the snotty, unfriendly people. So I headed back to a place that I once started to call *"home."* A place where *"anything goes;"* where natural ways were cool and where holistic healers were plentiful. I took the Amtrak train across the countryside -***Wow what a great trip !!*** It snowed in the mountains and was truly breathtaking. It was such a relaxing trip. It took me three days to get across the country, but it was well worth it. I had packed nine boxes and two suitcases as I headed west. I had my parents ship my car separately, which was also packed. I arrived in Sacramento on a cold January winter day in 1995; cold yes, but so refreshing. I knew this was where I was supposed to be, at least for the moment.

I stayed with a couple of friends till I found an apartment in Modesto, California, which is where I decided to call home. Having only the nine boxes, mainly cosmetics' inventory, computer stuff and my clothes, I had to buy everything else, which was ok by me ! It represented a wonderful new start in my world. I decided I was only going to buy what I liked and what felt good to me. So I chose leather furniture, brass and glass tables, accented by royal blue and emerald green colors. Over the next year or so, I added pieces to my collection to make it feel special and homier to me.

I continued to work for Beauti - Control Cosmetics and attempted to achieve directorship (a form of manage - ment), twice that year. I had never worked so hard, yet had so much fun in all my life. I got to help people look and feel their best through the use of this wonderfully color-coded make-up and skin care line, and taught them how to dress to feel like a million bucks – *even in a pair of jeans !* I was attempting to work the business full-time, but my major mood-swings got in my way, far too often.

I would run hard for a couple of weeks and then crash for three weeks, hardly moving off the couch. I would one minute have a wonderful attitude and purpose in life and the next be lying on the couch wishing I were dead. *The mood swings were quite severe – I could go from happy-go-lucky to depressed and angry in a matter of an hour !* I tried to cover it up, but those closest to me could see the swings quite vividly. When I was up and *"high"* on life, I felt like I could conquer the world and tried my best to do it. I had expanded my territory to eight states that year ! *I thought I was invincible – like no one or nothing could stop me !* **Boy was I wrong !**

Earlier that year, I was working on my computer, putting a newsletter to - gether for my team players, when all of a sudden I saw a glimpse of a bright light in the room. I was startled and kind of scared. I looked around to see if anyone was there, but I saw no one. Being reli - gious and feeling close to God, I quickly yelled out..."*Who are you and what do you want ? If you are good, you can stay, and if not then get the heck out of here,* **NOW** *!*"

I stood there waiting for something to happen and nothing did. So I returned to my computer and tried to continue working. Well whoever or whatever this bright light was, decided to play with me and turn the computer off on me, right before my eyes ! I was stunned and a bit upset (they forgot to save my work). I yelled again *"Who are you and what do you want.....??"*...**and still no answer.**

I decided I needed a break, so I left the computer off and went into my bed - room to pray and meditate. I asked God what was going on and who or what was this "being" and did they mean any harm to me. After sitting there quietly for a while which felt like eternity, I finally got an answer. I heard a voice say....

"We are angels and we are sent here by God to help you. We are going to teach you a lot about life, living, growing up and loving. There are seven of us and we mean no harm to you."

I was quickly relieved, but still a bit hesitant. I then fell asleep into a deep meditative state and felt much better upon rising. I returned to my computer work with a new energy and passion. All of a sudden I felt like I wasn't so alone any -

more, and that maybe God was really listening to all my prayers ! I had been asking for guidance, answers, teachers, healers, etc., to help me get well so I could be done with this recovery process. *Now I had seven of them ! THANK YOU GOD !*

During my quiet times, the angels would speak to me, mainly through my artwork, as they taught me how to paint on t-shirts. I would surrender to them late at night and allow them, while I was in meditation, to teach me to draw and paint-something I didn't know I could do. Each morning I would wake up and run into the dining room, where I had been laying the night before, to see what I had created. I was always in amazement

Here are a few pictures of my creative designs:

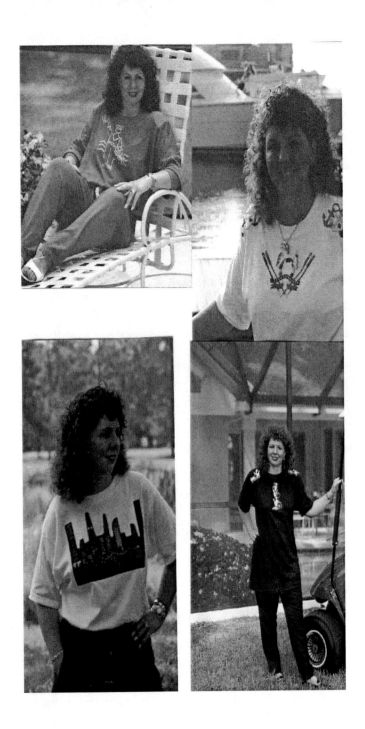

I learned to laugh that year - some - thing I had forgotten how to do. Being so depressed, yet intensely determined to get well, I had not lightened up on myself at all. I had forgotten the rule that you have to laugh at yourself or you will cry !

Even my newsletter and articles of inspiration for my team players changed that year. My team grew in leaps and bounds and everyone was growing stronger in their own businesses. I finally agreed to accept the challenge of director - ship, which was a huge career promotion for me if I could do it ! As I geared my team players up for this long 6-month trial period, I got stronger and better at leading them. I had grown in my business, not only as a strong manager and leader, but also as a glamour make-up artist and I loved it !! *I was one of the fastest make-up artists on the West Coast !* So I got to keep my wandering spirit happy by being able to travel to salons all over California and do glamour shots for women. Not only was

I making money and loving it, I was recruiting up a storm – which I needed for me to succeed to the next level.

Here are some glamour shots I had done for myself.

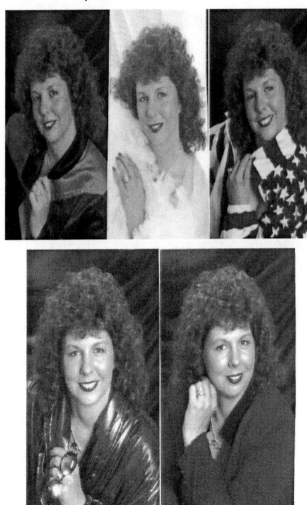

1995 was the year my *"adopted mom,"* and I reconnected. I call her my *"adopted mom,"* as she was a friend of my family for twenty years and was the closest *"mother figure"* to me at the time. She lived in Sacramento, which was only two hours away, and close enough to go visit. I had been told she was fighting cancer and going through a divorce. So I became her support team, and through our trying times and mood swings, we became great friends. She later decided to work with me in my clothing company and we are still close today. Since she was just up the road, I would go visit her frequently and it seemed to help both of us. We both needed each other as friends and as a support team. She was riding out cancer and a divorce, and I was riding the roller coaster of life, so we rode our journeys together.

I wanted this *"anniversary"* of my surgery to be special, so I got permission from my doctors to take scuba diving lessons – which I really wanted to do. I started dating a guy, who worked at a scuba shop, so I instantly had a dive buddy. I passed the class with flying colors and found a new activity I loved. It was so exciting, yet so peaceful underneath the water – no one could find me, bug me, call me or page me underwater – I felt so calm ! Finally some peace and quiet ! But even this temporary peace couldn't conquer my depression and mood swings !

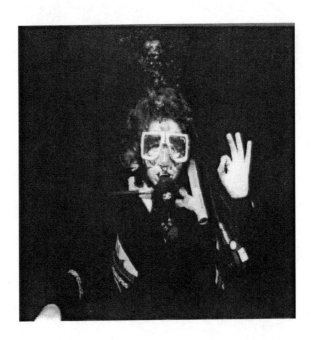

Unfortunately, I crashed! The depression got the best of me, and I didn't have the strength to get off that couch! As I struggled to keep the *"smiley face"* up and running for my team, but I was miserable inside. I was praying for a miracle every hour of every day, yet one never came. I was hoping some of my team players would help pick up the slack that month for me, but unfortunately, without my strength, motivation, and leadership, my team lost it's grip on the race for my promotion. I tried to re-group and get a positive attitude to try again, but I was so devastated and depressed, nothing helped or lasted long enough to make any difference!

My special surgery "anniversary" day is on the 13th of October and my real birthday is on November 6th – three weeks apart. As my real birthday crept upon me, I kept trying to get a grip on reality and find the real meaning to this word called *LIFE*. I saw several practitioners that year, including a psychotherapist, a nutritionist, a chiropractor, a psychic, and a preacher. All of a sudden, all of my motivational talks and thoughts didn't mean a thing anymore and I was falling deeper and deeper into depression. I really was escaping into a fantasy world, because reality was too tough ! I wanted to believe that if I could just settle down, fall in love and get married, I would become *"normal,"* but that never happened !

The Christmas season was once again upon me and I had very little spirit. My business had almost completely died and I had no energy or spunk for gift baskets or open houses. My parents came to town right when I was emotionally ex - hausted. My mom and I got into a car accident 5 days before Christmas that year and that was the last straw that pushed me over the edge.

On December 25th – late at night, I was in total pain from the injuries and couldn't sleep, even though I had taken some pain pills. So I got up, packed my bags and decided I was going to run away and leave California for good. So I stuffed things into my suitcases thinking I would never return and might even have to sleep in my car a bit. Packed and ready to go, I took off driving, telling no one where I was going, cause I really didn't know myself. I drove west over the mountains and valley areas and finally at 3 AM pulled into a little motel to sleep; not really knowing how far I had driven or where I was I retiring for the night. Upon waking I was in extreme pain, out-of-town, not knowing anyone and not even knowing where I was - *boy was I scared !!* I called my best friend in South Carolina and I even scared her. She finally convinced me to go to the front desk and ask where I was and where I could find a doctor. I found out I was in Marina, California and I guessed that meant near the ocean, but that was all it meant at that time. Little did I realize I was near

Monterey, California – a place I now call *"heaven on earth."*

I finally called a referral service and found a doctor. Upon meeting him I found out I had 4 broken ribs, internal bleeding and no recollection how I did this ! By now, my mom and the accident was just a blurr. Now according to him I could only walk or lay, with absolutely no sitting. (It hurt to sit anyway). He gave me some pain pills and told me to stay in town for the New Year's weekend. *Boy, I was not only bummed, but very scared !!* Since I had to walk a lot, I soon discovered this wonder - ful town. My parents finally found out where I was and, as usual, were upset with me again and my *"irrational and childish"* behavior. Little did they or I realize this *"irrational"* episode of mine would soon help me find my next town to live in. I finally called a girlfriend, who with her son, came over, got me and drove me home. I stayed home for a week or two and decided to return to the Monterey area to inquire about moving there. Upon returning there the second time, I really saw the beauty and serenity in the town, which inspired me to move there. I located a one - bedroom apartment, five blocks from the ocean and returned home to start packing. Because I was starting out brand new again, I resigned from BeautiControl. I also decided to continue to see my boy - friend, but the distance made it harder and more infrequent.

Once packed and loaded, I chose to fly my best friend from South Carolina out to see California, help me unpack and spend some quality time together. For a week we toured all over the Bay area, exploring new places as we went along. I made these decisions at that time, know - ing my financial freedom was soon coming to a screeching halt, as I was planning on filing bankruptcy that spring. I realized I was way over my head in debt and couldn't see the light of day to get out of it. Because I had charged a lot of my cosmetics to my credit cards, and then bought impulsively through my various mood swings, I was overwhelmed with bills I knew I couldn't pay.

Moving to Monterey was one of the neatest and most rewarding moves in this lifetime. The angels were right there every step of the way, guiding me, teaching me, laughing and crying with me.

Here are some pictures of the beautiful coastline.

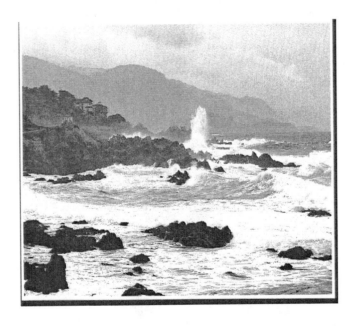

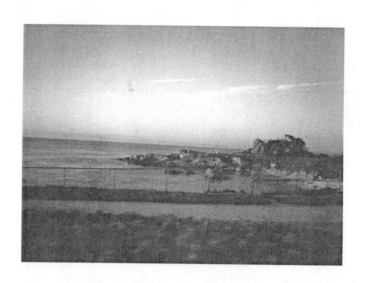

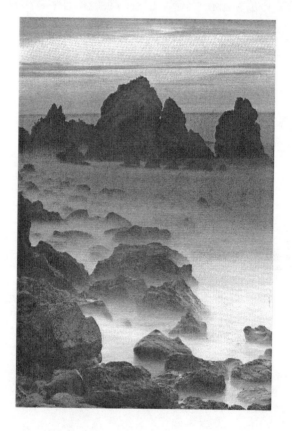

In February 1996, I finally got to "see" my angels and they were so beauti-ful... *all seven of them* ! They were small in size, but very angelic and graceful looking. They looked a lot like what people call **"cherubs"** today. They came to me in a dream and told me I was going to start designing clothes for a living ! I almost laughed, as I didn't like to sew, and wasn't a professional artist either ! I didn't really believe in my artistic talent and could not see this happening at all. So I asked for some confirmation from them and over the next seven days, I had total strangers tell me the outfits that I had made and wore were gorgeous and asked me what boutique did I buy them in ! On the seventh day, my angels came to me and said – *"well do you believe us now ?"* I agreed. So with them by my side, guiding me every step of the way, I started my own clothing company called *The Added Touch – Clothing with Added Flair, later re-named Acaysha – Clothing With An Added Touch.*

I worked hard to create many new designs, as I prepared to participate in a health and holistic trade show in three weeks. I called on my *"adopted mom"* to help me get started and she was delighted. She was still struggling with cancer and a divorce, so this gave her something to do and helped take her mind off her pro - blems. She cut out the appliques and designs as I created each and every outfit by hand. My best friend in South Carolina decided she wanted to become part of this project too, so she jumped in also and helped me in the cutting department. I did the show, learned a lot, sold a little and met many new people and contacts. Luckily, I knew how to do trade shows from my cosmetic days so networking was easy for me. I took a few orders and hurried home to fill them and contact others.

Unfortunately, the depression kept sneaking up on me and knocking me for a loop, but this time I continued to perse -

vere and work at this new venture. I finally got enough designs put together, that I was able to ask some friends to model for me while a professional photographer took pictures so I could make a catalog. They were delighted, and the photo shoot went well. I then developed the photos and soon learned how to make my own catalog. I designed the cover, the introduction, the price sheets, the items and their names, the numbers and everything...*boy, what a new and exhilarating challenge !* I finally got the first copy of the catalog together and made a plan to go to Nashville in August for a cosmetic convention and sell my wears there !

As my creativity continued, new and exciting designs came into being. Every - one was enjoying this venture; both of my best friends, one in South Carolina and one in Sacramento, California, were help - ing me get this company off the ground. Little did I realize how much was involved in manufacturing clothing. My father had been in the food manufacturing industry all of his life, but this was so different. We were just a small 3 women operation, trying to compete against the *"big boys !"* The details that went into designing the label, the catalog, the artwork, the adver - tising, the marketing, the recruiting and hiring of others, were **overwhelming**. Boy, little did I see the whole picture to this venture, and my father was too busy in his career to give me business advice or guidance. *But I was willing to learn and with this team of seven angels, I was willing to try anything !*

During this season, the angels finally let me paint them so others could see them too. *Boy were they beautiful !* As I sat at the computer trying to come up with traditional angel names for them – I heard one angel say, *"that's not my name !"* I was shocked, but more comfortable with them, I replied, *"Oh, so what is your name ?"* I was expecting any one of many names, but not the one she typed. She erased what I had typed and typed... _Childs Play_. I was stunned, I said _"that's not an angel name,"_ for which she quickly responded, _"okay, but that is my name !"_ She said she was here to **teach me to laugh, cry and play – just like a kid and to learn to love my "inner child."**

She was my _"three-year old child."_ Boy was I in for a lot of great adventures with her. She was the most outspoken of them all, and the funniest. _She would make me do crazy things like eat a candy bar, put my feet in the sand at the beach and ride with the windows down (when it was 50 de - grees outside!)... crazy, but fun-spirited things !_ I learned to live again through her. She helped me give names to all the other angels too, none of them like I would have named them.

During all of this, I was meeting new and exciting people, many in the holistic field. I found a wonderful group of like-minded people at a get-together one night and they soon became my _"spiritual_ *family."* I began to learn who I really was, where I came from, and what I was here to do. I took many classes that year and learned many news skills and techniques on how to heal myself. They ranged from rolfing to numerology to crystal healings to general spirituality. *I was like a sponge... I wanted to learn everything !! Anything that would help me heal, ease the pain and grow-up, I was game to learn ! I also learned how to laugh (I already knew how to cry) and "live in the moment" that summer.*

I became very active in this spiritual group of seekers and soon felt like I had found a place I could really call *"home,"* with people I could trust. I felt more con - nected to these people than I did my own family. These people seemed to under - stand what I was dealing with and encour - aged me to grow and experience along the way. I felt like I was finally getting my depression under my control. I proceeded to file for bankruptcy and it went through without any problems – *I was finally debt free !!*

During that summer, I decided to go on a spiritual vacation to Hawaii and swim with dolphins. I had heard that dolphins are healing animals and I was willing to try anything to get well. So I read all I could get my hands on about dolphins and their healing abilities. I could hardly wait because I just knew they would help me get well ! I went with a girlfriend and we had a ball ! On our fourth day, we got to swim with them – *out in the wild blue ocean ! Talk about exciting !!* When we got out of the boat and into the water, everyone headed for shore, except me. I could not see what they were following, and just then I saw something out of the corner of my eye. So I headed that way, which was towards the open ocean ! *Seven dolphins* soon surrounded me and they were guiding me out to the middle of the Pacific Ocean ! I couldn't touch them because they were just out of my range, but they were so breathtaking, I didn't care. I couldn't believe I had seven dolphins all to myself. Then, *all of a sudden, they disappeared into the bottom of the ocean and I stopped swimming. I looked up and couldn't see anything or anyone. I finally saw a small white dot in the far distance, and I assumed that was the boat.... oh well, I thought. Guess I'll just have to swim back ! At least I was a good swimmer ! I started to snorkel back and all of a sudden the dolphins re-appeared and guided me back to the boat !! Oh what a thrill !!* I took some pictures, because in my mind I was thinking no one would believe that I had seven dolphins of my own. I thought, *"Boy, I hope they would make an appearance,"* and as soon as I got my feet on the ladder and was safely back on the boat, they individually jumped over the bough of the boat. *Everyone was ecstatic and cheering with joy !* After talking about my experi-ence, I started to draw them in my notebook and to write my messages and feelings down. I was elated and felt blessed and healed. When we went to group discussion that evening, I talked a lot and everyone was tickled with my stories. Here are some of the pictures I took while there:

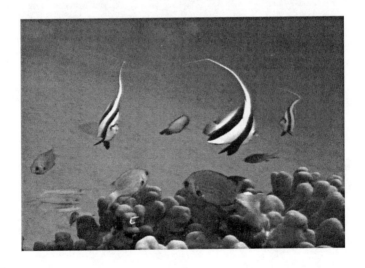

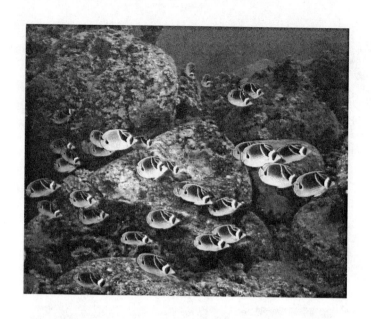

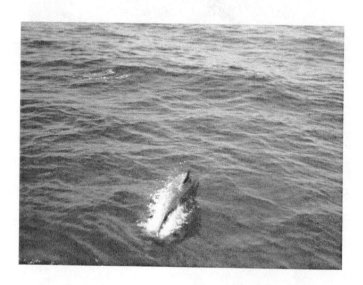

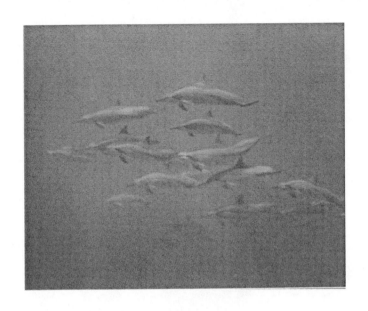

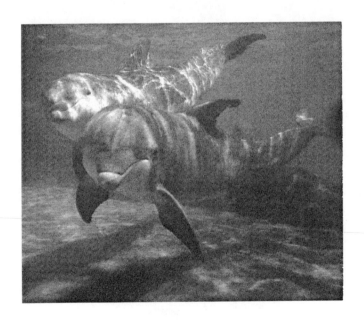

Here is one of the songs I wrote
after my encounter with the dolphins:

SONG I HEARD IN MY SLEEP IN KONA, HAWAII - DEDICATED FROM MY ANGELS TO MY DOLPHIN SPIRIT GROUP

ANGELS AMONG US
ANGELS SURROUND US

WE COME TO TEACH YOU,
GUIDE YOU AND LOVE YOU

ANGELS AMONG US
ANGELS SURROUND US

WE'RE HERE TO SUPPORT YOU
AND SHOW YOU THE WAY

ANGELS AMONG US
ANGELS SURROUND US

WE SHOW UP IN MANY
FORMS, SHAPES AND TONES

SO PLEASE LET US GUIDE YOU,
LOVE YOU AND TEACH YOU
SO THAT YOU CAN GROW
TO LEVELS BEYOND.

Upon returning home from Hawaii, I proceeded to make dolphins my main focus in my designs and the number one selling item in my entire line. Here are some pictures of the new designs I created.

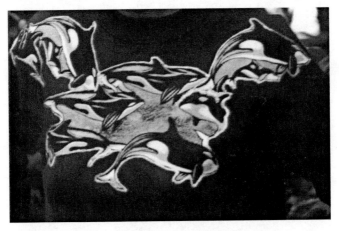

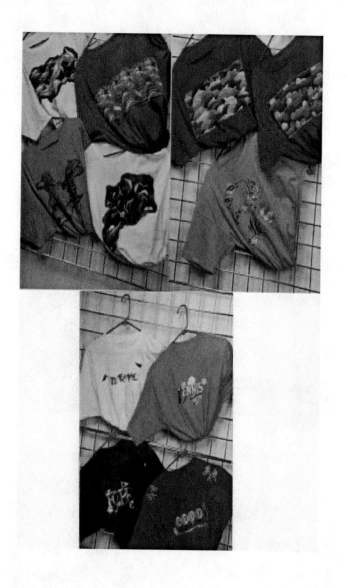

I proceeded to get ready for the Nashville trip, only to come home and find out I was pregnant (and I was on the pill). I told my boyfriend, hoping it would be good news, but he wasn't happy and said only that he would help raise it but not marry me. I took the news in stride, and shared it quietly with a few close friends. My new *"family"* of friends was ecstatic, saying I must be caring an angel, since I got pregnant while on the pill. That made me feel a little better.

I unfortunately miscarried the child and in looking for comfort and condo - lences, I called my mom. Unfortunately, she was very upset and proceeded to preach at me for getting pregnant in the first place. *I was devastated !!* I was looking for a friend and found only an enemy. That was the beginning of a very long struggle for my life, especially with my mom.

As my body started to cry out in mourning and agony, I couldn't eat or keep food down; my head was dizzy and all my major organs began to shut down. By the time I made an appointment to see the healers in town, *I was 80% shut down and almost dead.* While working on me, they told me I had to make a decision whether I wanted to stay here on the planet or go home, but before I made that decision, an angel would like to speak to me. I agreed to listen, and as the angel spoke I realized it was **Childs Play**, and she said,

*"Mommy, I want you to know it wasn't your fault. I needed to learn a lesson in grounding before I could come to the planet. **You did no wrong !!** You are welcome to come home and we will wel - come you with open arms, but I would love for you to stay, as one day I will be yours to have and to hold. But I can only come back if you stay on the planet and do your mission work."*

Then she was gone. With tears in my eyes, I agreed to stay and I felt my soul come back into my body. Upon finishing my healing session I thanked my friends and went home to rest. I shed many tears in the next few days, as I released the emptiness from within. Even though my heart felt a little better, my depression was still keeping a tight hold on me.

Not long after that encounter with the angel, I decided to bring Raffaella into my world. Raffaella was a kitten; a pure bred Persian with silver markings and green eyes. I had never had a cat before, because in my younger years I was allergic to them. But my spiritual friends, who raised them, insisted I needed someone to care for and someone to share my love with. Knowing nothing about raising cats, I proceeded to read a lot and ask lots of questions. *Raffaella was a great joy in my life, someone I could give love to, cuddle with and care for.* Raffaella was like an angel, a healing angel at that, as she would lie on my chest and just purr, sending me much love and light.

Isn't she beautiful ?

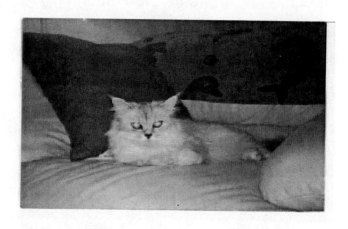

In October of that year, I returned to
Arizona to see the doctors, hoping to get
this depression thing under control.
Unfortunately, I was so down and out, that
I wrote a suicide note to my doctor, saying
*"If they sent me home telling me every -
thing was **"fine,"** that I would guarantee
them I would be dead by the weekend."* The
suicide letter took them by surprise, and
they decided to keep me for three weeks
to observe me.

During that time I wrote a prayer
type poem, explaining my frustration and
fears.

This Prayer/Poem Was Written on
October 12, 1996,
One Day Before My
4-year anniversary

WHY DOES IT HAVE TO BE SO HARD ??

I just want to forgive and let go.
I just want to forgive and let go.

I don't want to deal,
I don't want to deal anymore.
I don't want to fight; I do not want to fight.
I'm tired and stressed too far
And I don't want to fight anymore.

I just want to forgive and forget.
I just want to forgive and let go,
But it keeps coming back;
It keeps coming back !
I don't want to fight anymore !

I just want to live and go forward.
I'm tired of dying and going backwards.

I just want to forgive and let go.
I just want to forget and go on.

I just want to leave; I just want to leave;
I just want to leave and let go.

I don't have the strength to go on.
I don't have the strength to go on.
It doesn't get easier; it only gets harder.
I just want to forgive and let go.

I don't see a purpose to go on.
I don't see a purpose to go on.
It used to seem great to go on,
But I'm tired and worn and I
Just want to forgive and let go.

I don't want to deal anymore.
I've only been going from crisis to crisis.
I don't want to deal anymore.

I thought it would be easier after surgery.
I thought I had a chance
To be "normal" but it only got harder.
It only got harder.

I thought it would get easier after this.
I just want to leave and be gone.
I just want to leave and be gone.
Even if I come back; even if I have
To come back, it's got to be
Easier than this.
I just want to forgive and let go.
I just want to forgive and let go.

Why does it have to be so hard ?
Why can't I do it easier ?
What did I do to deserve all of this ?
What did I do so bad to deserve all of this
At such an early age ?

Why continue ? – to go from one crisis to
another forever ? **NOT !!**
My tools for dealing are few.
My tools for leaving are many !
Please give me a break to regroup
And ground.
I've tried and I've tried !

I just want to forgive and let go !
I just want to forget and let go !

I spoke to the psychiatrist many times, with only small successes. Between visits, I shopped a lot, walked around the hotel and then something unexpected happen.

I met a wonderful young man, who raised my heart and my mind off all my worries. We began to see each other almost every day while I was in town, and as expected, my mood swings picked up. You see, I am a people person and need to have people in my world, who love me and care for me and at this time in my life, I really needed someone to love me. He was a roofer who was starting up his business in the area. He gave me the attention and affection I so badly needed and desired !

Then the doctors decided I was fine and could return home to California. I was hesitant to leave, as I didn't want this dream to end. I promised I would come visit frequently and he said he would try too and then I got on the plane and re - turned home to California. Right away I was missing him badly because I really was lacking in love and attention in my life.

I wanted to go back to Arizona immediately, but then he called and said he was coming for a visit. I eagerly went to the airport to pick him up and our visit was great. I showed him all over the Monterey peninsula and when it came time for him to leave I didn't want him to go. He asked me what my thoughts were regarding him starting his business in the area. I was stunned and ecstatic all at the same time, as that would mean I would get to see him a lot more. So he decided to open his roofing business in Monterey, and I was on *cloud nine.*

Life seemed so much better that fall, as I had someone to care for and someone who loved me back. I just kept praying that my dream life would soon get started...then I could be *"normal."* He started to get a couple of roofing jobs in the area, and I was helping him with the marketing of the company.

That Christmas, he proposed to me, *he asked me to marry him, and I eagerly said "Yes !!"* We went to the San Francisco wholesale market to get my ring; one I got to pick out and have designed. It was gorgeous. I was floating on a cloud much higher than number nine. We went home to New Jersey for Christmas that year and that was when my dream life came to a screeching halt. My parents didn't like him and obviously the feelings were mutual, so upon our return to California, we started fighting and bickering a lot...something I wasn't used to and didn't like at all. I tried so hard to make everything right, but it just got worse and we finally broke up. *I was heart broken, angry and devastated. I was overrun with feelings ! I so much wanted it to work, but no matter how much talking we did, nothing seemed to help.* I decided to move to another area and a new home, as the memories were driving me crazy and I also needed more room for the clothing business.

*Do I seem like a fast moving person to you ? **Well I am !** I was on a mission. I wanted to be "normal, and healthy," quickly ! I would do **anything, I mean any - thing under the sun and stars to get well - as long as it was natural, and it didn't involve drugs or surgery !!** I still am a* ***"mover and a shaker"*** *type* person, as life is too short to let it pass me by.

    "Grab it by the horns and don't let go ! Live life to the fullest, each and every day. Live it like it is your first and last day and don't go to bed mad, angry or regretful !" Those are words I live by.

    I decided upon coming out of my surgery, that I was going to live by those words and I was going to do everything in my power to get well and be healthy for the latter part of my life. I made that promise to God on those Red Rocks in Sedona – that I would do whatever he/she wanted me to do in this lifetime; if he/she let my surgery be a success, I would do what I was meant to do down here for

him/her. I would work for God for the rest
of my life.

THE DREAMER AND THE HEALER - CH.6

In January, 1997,I found a large 3
bedroom duplex house for rent in the
town next door to Monterey called Salinas
"the lettuce capital" of the world. I moved
myself, taking several trips back and forth,
becoming exhausted while I was burning
the candle at both ends. I was trying to
move, pack, unpack and keep my clothing
business alive all at the same time. The
house had an add-on living room and extra
bedroom, kind of like an in-law quarters,
which served as my production studio for
the clothing.

I was still in a huge learning curve
that year, as I took several classes in
numerology, crystals, hypnosis, astrology,
and channeling and became a Reiki
Master. Reiki is a universal healing energy,
the same that Jesus used in his days to
heal people. It is unconditional love and
warmth that moves through a *"laying on of
hands"* healing technique. I was game to

learn anything that could possibly get me well, as long as it didn't include drugs or surgery ! I would try anything at this point to be healthy and kick this depression. I was even attending church, hoping the sermons would help find new strength and hope to keep moving forward !

I was also given my new spiritual name, which I go by today, **_Acaysha,_** **_which means angel of diversity and_** **_strength,_** _and after reading this book, you_ _will agree with it !!_ My spiritual teachers said everyone has a spiritual name. Although not given to us by our parents at birth, it is really who we are. It took me almost 2 more years to finally get used to my name and use it comfortably around the masses. I first used my name only in spiritual circles and around like-minded individuals. But after many more experi - ences in this lifetime, I had finally realized that I had a different personality in this body kinda like a _"walk-in"_ and the two-personalities had finally merged into one, which is who I am today.

Raffaella really liked her new home, as we had a fenced in the backyard where she could lie out in the sun and enjoy the fresh air. I tried to mate her that year, but she didn't like the *"stud muffin"* I chose for her. Since he was a stud for hire, she wanted nothing to do with him !

I was trying to understand diet, food combinations and how to lose weight the right way this year also, so I became a very strict vegetarian, to the point of no eggs, chicken, fish or dairy - a vegan vegetarian. *Boy was this routine a tough one !* I wanted to lose weight the proper way, but I was having no success. The dietitian I was seeing could not understand why I was having no luck in dropping the pounds. I later found out my metabolism was "dead," my thyroid was not working, my adrenals were still shot from my re - covery, and that diet pills were needed to help the metabolism get jump-started.

After many long days and nights alone and much fluctuation in my income level, I decided to return to the working force, outside of the home. I needed daily people contact or I was going to go crazy. I actually checked myself into the psych - iatric ward of Stanford Hospital for eight days, before starting back to work !! They put me on Depakote to balance my moods and bi-polar swings. It seemed to make a real difference, *at least for a little while.* It was the same drug I was on when I came out of surgery and had been on for years as an epileptic, so my body was used to it. Even the doctors there felt that going out into the workforce was a good idea.

A mass-merchandising chain was getting ready to open a new store in our area and I had never opened a store in my retail career, so this sounded like a new and exciting adventure to me. I applied and got hired in June of 1997. We worked 80-hour weeks for almost six months. I was exhausted, but was loving the thrill of it – *talk about a high !* I did very well and got promoted within the first few months of opening of the store.

Unfortunately, in November of that year, I had an accident and fell eight feet off a ladder. I was hurt pretty badly, as I landed on my feet, jamming my spine from the bottom up and impacted my left arm while trying to catch myself ! But it was a week before Thanksgiving and I knew better than to call in sick, so I kept working, no matter how much pain I was in !

After several trips to the chiro - practor and massage person, I felt a bit better. That Christmas was a busy one, yet very lonely. Because I was working so many hours, I had no time to go back to see my family, so I spent it alone with laryngitis and bronchitis. My doctors wanted me to slow down, but I didn't know how. *The constant running kept my de - pression at bay, as I had no time to feel or be low.*

Unfortunately, in February of 1998 I got hurt again, this time worse than be - fore ! *I had a computer desk fall off a shelf and hit me on my head, right across my surgery scar line !* **OUCH** *!!* This movement jammed everything from the top of my neck down to the bottom of my spine and did in both arms and shoulders too. Within a week, I couldn't even stand up straight ! I got written off work and the doctors tried to give me pain pills. Un - fortunately I was allergic to almost all the drugs on the market, so the pain pill, daypro that they gave me, made me hallucinate. I hallucinated for almost a week, before I convinced a friend to drive me to Stanford Hospital to be reviewed.

My friend didn't like to drive, little did I know, so she asked her ex-husband to take us both, and he did. He sat by my side the whole eight hours I was in the emergency room and finally after several blood tests and exams, they finally gave me something to bring me back into my body. *What an experience !* After that I decided to get a lawyer to represent me and protect me regarding this accident case.

The interesting twist to this story was that the ex-husband and I became really close friends and finally started dating each other because of this event. He would call or come by almost daily to check on me and make sure I was doing ok. I really appreciated the attention and was starting to fall for him.

I decided I didn't want to go back to work for this employer anymore. Two accidents was enough for me in this lifetime ! After a month of staying home and re - covering, I applied for a position in outside sales in another town. Before starting my new job and making the move to another town, my father's company, to celebrate his retirement, flew me into Arizona. My brother and I were the *"surprise guests"* for his retirement party, *boy was he shocked to see us !* After returning home from the

163

retirement party I decided to move closer to work and my boyfriend decided to join me, scared to let me move that far away without him. So we moved to a town in the East Bay of California. It was a commuter town for sure; surrounded by freeways. I started my new job, only to realize I was not cut out for door knocking and outside sales. *I definitely was a new person; the old me loved the challenge of door knocking and getting the sales, while this new person I had become did not !* I didn't last long in the outside sales world, so I decided to return to what I knew best, retail management.

I got a job as an assistant manager in a high-class retail chain store. It was a great store offering everything for today's woman, from shorts and t-shirts, to suits and evening gowns and all the accessories to match. It brought my entire image con - sulting experience to a new level !

During this time I became engaged to this guy and was trying to plan a wedding. He had met my parents and asked my father for my hand in marriage, my father consented. Both of my parents seemed to like him; *this was a first in my life.* This was an extremely stressful time for both of us - new to the town, adjusting to new bosses and circumstances, trying to plan a wedding and still find time to laugh and love. The stress got to both of us and we broke off the engagement in the summer, trying to re-group our thoughts and feelings. I decided to join Mary Kay cosmetics, because of a neat lady I met at our store. She convinced me to go to Dallas for the convention to get a com - plete picture of the company. I agreed.

Obviously I wasn't supposed to be working in retail, as I got hurt on this job too. *(Murphy's law, I guess !!) I had a metal bar fall on my head, while trying to do a floor move and that put me out of work for over 2 years !!* But as you always hear, there is good in everything, no matter how bad it might appear ! However, my throbbing head and I were starting to wonder about that phrase.

Since we had broken up, my ex-fiancé told me to go date others and let him have his space. I was reluctant to do this at first but then I met a great guy on the Internet. He lived in Texas, so I decided to meet him when I went out there for the Mary Kay conference. He was a great guy, with wonderful values, and morals, but my heart was torn between taking a chance with him or going back to California and working it out with my ex-fiancé. I chose the later. Upon returning to California, I started to pursue my career with Mary Kay, but I just didn't have the drive I used to have in my days with BeautiControl Cosmetics. Besides, unfor - tunately I was allergic to the line, so I didn't last long with the company !

My ex-fiancé and I got re-engaged again in late July and he decided to pursue his dreams in the aviation industry. *I had always told him to follow his dreams, no* *matter where they would lead him, with or without me. **Life was too short to be miserable, and I still believe that !*** He went to school to learn to be an aviation mechanic, fixing and maintaining air - planes.

JOURNEY BACK TO THE SOUTH;
THE WEIGHT LOSS SUCCESS STORY
CHAPTER 7

It was during all of these changes that I was seeing another dietitian in the area, still trying to get my weight off. I was now a heavy size 14, almost a 16, the heaviest I had ever been; a whopping 259 pounds !! It was during this time in July I found a wonderful new company called *Trek* that was marketing a new all-natural diet pill. I had never taken diet pills before, as I believed you had to do it through the food you ate, not through a drug or pill. *But, being reluctant yet desperate, I decided to try it, as I was destined to be a bride in 9 months !* I was told to take my measurements, weight and take some pictures so I would know where I started. Those statistics were more than I wanted to know at the time, but I did it. Weighing in at 259 lbs. with hips measuring 44 1/2 inches, my bra size was a 38DD. I didn't need much more information to convince me to at least try these pills for 30 days as they came with a 30-day money back guarantee. *I decided to give them a shot and within 21 days I had dropped 20 pounds! I was ecstatic !!*

My dietitian couldn't believe they were working for me, but at that point I didn't care, because the pounds needed to come off. So I decided to stay on them and see if I could get all my weight off. *By Christmas that year, I had lost 60 pounds and was wearing a size 8 !* I have an hour-glass shape; so I lost weight in every inch of my body, including my feet.... they shrunk ½ a shoe size !

That fall after my fiancé completed his schooling, we moved across the country to Greensboro, North Carolina, where he got a start in his new career. Being hurt, off work and engaged I de - cided to move with him and start a new life together. We were able to buy a house, with the help of nice down payment from my parents, an early wedding present they said. We moved in on Halloween weekend and I had less than three weeks to get the house in order, as his parents were coming down from West Virginia for Thanksgiving to meet me. I did it, thanks to my wonderful angels and their help. His parents really liked me and my parents liked him; everything seemed like it was going well. I think my parents were just glad to see me settling down with some - one and be back in the Carolinas, closer to them !

That Christmas season came and went pretty smoothly and I decided to return to college, as I was bored and wanted something to do. My employer was going to have to re-train me any way, so I decided to go back to college and finish my marketing degree, *once and for all !!*

I started back in January at the University of North Carolina at Greensboro and loved it ! I needed a new challenge, now that the house was set-up, and

because he worked second shift. Unfortunately, he began to feel inadequate and
inferior to me as I pursued my education,
as he thought I would leave him when I got
my degree. This was the furthest thing
from my mind, as I was so happy to be
engaged and looking forward to being
married in a few months. He felt I would
run off with a young 18 year-old boy, even
though I was 32 years old and wore an
engagement ring on my finger !

This insecurity of his caused major
problems in our relationship and he finally
pushed me too far, causing me to have an
anxiety attack whereupon I ended up in
the emergency room that night at 4 AM.
My parents drove up from Hilton Head,
South Carolina the next day and asked me
what I wanted to do to correct the
situation. Not thinking very clearly at that
time because they had pumped Valium
into my system to stop the anxiety attack,
my answer was *"I want him out of my life
and I mean now !"* So within 24 hours we

put the house on the market and pro -
ceeded to sell it in less than 24 days ! *With*
less than 2 months left before our wedd -
ing date, I was back to being single, un-
engaged, alone and scared, and in a town I
didn't really want to be in ! I was strugg -
ling to keep my grades up in school, while
trying to see the light of day through my
hurt feelings. He and I broke up and then
didn't speak for months.

I was trying to find balance and
peace in my world but now I had my
parents telling me I should *"move home,"*
or *"move closer to home."* I was fighting
the thought of being controlled by anyone,
especially my parents ! After my New
Jersey incidents in '94, I decided not to
move home ever again ! I think I deal
better with my family and their problems
when I live further away. I don't want to be
"down the street" from them, *EVER* !!

My anxiety attacks were many and I
was back under a Counselor's care. I finally
finished my semester at school and decid -

ed to hit the road and travel for my clothing business. I was on the road for 7 weeks that summer, going from trade show to trade show. I did Dallas, New York, Charlotte, and Fort Lauderdale, Florida.

Between the Charlotte and Fort Lauderdale show I got news that my father was going to have surgery, as they thought he might have prostate cancer. I was horrified, scared, and mad all in the same breath. I went down to Hilton Head, South Carolina to visit him and to hear the details of this condition. *To my amaze - ment, he was going to have a laser treat - ment that would only take 30 minutes, yet he was convinced he was going to die !* Boy did I find out how little compassion I had for him. *He was afraid of a 30-minute laser surgery and I went through an 8- hour brain surgery !!* I wasn't buying this, so I told him I loved him and would support him, but I wasn't going to sit around and help him waddle in his pain and misery. Especially since he didn't have any compassion for me all those years with my epilepsy. ***"Take 2 pills and go back to work,"*** was his phrase to me all those years - now it was my turn to give him the same lecture. The laser surgery didn't work and they proceeded to do 3 more surgeries to get it right. I showed up for the first one, but again I had no patience with the whining and moaning part. He did say, ***"I deserve this don't I ?"*** I agreed. The fourth surgery was finally a success and he didn't have cancer, thank God !

As I left for the Fort Lauderdale show, my mom assured me that he was fine. Upon arriving in Fort Lauderdale, I fell in love with the ocean scene; the fresh air and the warm summer nights. You see my arm was still hurting from all of those work-related accidents, which happened over a year ago. I was almost paralyzed, to the point where brushing my hair was a daily challenge ! Then while being in Florida, I was enjoying the warm summer nights along the beach front, when I noticed I hadn't taken any pain pills (herbal) or used my heating pad at all while I was there. *I was ecstatic !!*

Upon returning to the Carolinas, I went into deep pain and depression. I decided the cold damp weather was not helping my condition and questioned my - self as to why I was staying there. I had no real reason anymore because originally, I had only moved there to support my ex-fiancé and his new career move, expecting at that time to end up happily married !

By designing my own clothing line out of my home, I could live anywhere I chose. I decided to return to Florida to see if the weather really had something to do with my pain remission or not, or *discover it was just a lucky break; a temporary miracle in my life.* Upon crossing the state line I began to feel better. I drove all over the state looking at places and towns to live in, finally deciding on the Fort Lauder - dale area where my original miracle had occurred. Next, I found an apartment and drove home determined to pack and move, *again !*

I proceeded to gather up my belongings and move south, only to be detoured by Hurricane Floyd ! I stopped in Hilton Head to see my parents, just in time to be facing the 100 mile per hour incoming rains and winds from the ever-present hurricane. We left and went inland to a small town in Georgia. Once the storm passed, I left my parents and headed south as they returned back to Hilton Head. After several obstacles and inconveniences, I finally got settled into my apartment in Sunrise, Florida, in the fall of 1999.

During all of this I continued to lose more weight ! Here is the story I had written about my weight loss success:

ACAYSHA LANNING'S SUCCESS STORY
WITH BIO-ENERGETIC

I started taking Bio-Energetic in July
'98, right after I got proposed to. I was 259
pounds wearing a size 14 (I'm only 5'3). I am
an hourglass shape and I gain weight EVERY-
WHERE, including my feet, my fingers, my
face, my arms - **everywhere !!** I knew I had to
buy wedding gown 2 sizes bigger than I was -
meaning a size 18 ! No way was I going to do
that. I had been under the direction of 2
different dieticians in the last 2 years and no -
thing had seemed to work. I had tried eating
once a day, three times a day, even five times
a day. I had gone strictly vegetarian, no
chicken or fish - just vegetables, tofu, rice, and
some fruits ! I was walking 2 - 5 miles a day,
working out (I had re-joined another gym in
May '98), drinking my water, etc and nothing
was getting the weight off !! Everyone,

including my nutritionists, were all frustrated and dumbfounded. **Nothing seemed to work that would allow me to drop the weight !** Wanting to change jobs I saw an ad for sales in health and beauty so I called on it - this is how I found Trek Alliance and was introduced to the Bio-Energetic weight loss products.

I said I would try the product for 30 days with the Money Back Guarantee and I wanted cash on the 29th day if it didn't work ! **I didn't believe it would work because nothing else did** and only if it did work would I be interested in selling it. **So skeptically, I tried it, not expecting to see any results.** I weighed and measured before I started: 259 pounds, my bra size was a 38DD my hips were 44 1/2," my waist was 32" and my bust measured 41 1/4". **Boy did I need to lose**

**weight badly and quickly - I was due to
marry April '99 !!**

So I did everything I was told to do -
taking a total of 4 pills a day, 2 in the mid-
morning, 2 in mid-afternoon. I was still eating
right, with fish, chicken, vegetables, etc in my
diet. About 3 weeks into this, I noticed my bra
was not fitting right. Then I stepped on the
scales - it said I had **lost 20 pounds !!** Not
believing it I asked my fiancé to step on them.
He never gained any weight and he said they
were accurate.

I was SHOCKED; yet EXCITED !!

He said he had noticed a change too
and he encouraged me to stay on it ! So I
decided to stay on them to see if I had finally
found something that was going to work for
me. I started dropping weight pretty quickly

and by Christmas '98, I was wearing a size 8 and was 60 pounds lighter.

By March '99 I was in a size 6 and 80 pounds down ! I stayed a size 6 most of that year. Having an hourglass shaped body, I had to lose from every inch of my body to see a difference, but I was still very muscular from my sport days as a teen. On my body, 10 pounds could be one dress size, depending where I lost the weight from ! **By January 1, 2000, I was wearing a size 4 in some of my clothes !** I had dropped another 40 pounds over the holiday season, due to me dealing with the cancer news I received at Thanks - giving time !

I am now comfortably wearing between a size 4 and 6, depending on the designer and am holding my own at 120 pounds lighter ! With measurements of a bra size 36C, (haven't worn a C since I was 16 !) my hips are now 34 3/8", waist 24 1/2", and breast 35" ! I did not exercise during this time, (except casual walking) as I had been hurt on the job and was not allowed to exercise until summer 2000.

So all my success goes to **Trek Alliance** and their wonderful Bio-energetic diet pills ! I have another 22 pounds to go (upper thighs) and then I will be done.

From July '98 till now my life has been hectic: I got hurt on the job, got engaged, made a move from California to North Carolina, bought a house, and then sold the house 4 months later when I broke my engagement. Then I moved into an apartment in NC and finally relocated to Fort Lauderdale, Florida in Sept '99, right after Hurricane Floyd. Then I returned to College to finish my *marketing degree, while working 40 hours a week and dealing with cancer !*

Now that I have dropped my weight - I feel great and look FANTASTIC. Many friends say I look younger now and my single life is flourishing again ! With all these trying times and stresses - I still managed to keep my weight off and kept losing more pounds too !
If I can do it with all of this going on then you can too !

I have enclosed some before and after pictures for your enjoyment. Hope this story encourages you to take control of your weight problem for the last and final try ! I took the chance and it worked for me. I wish you much success in your future and may your weight just drop off, like mine !

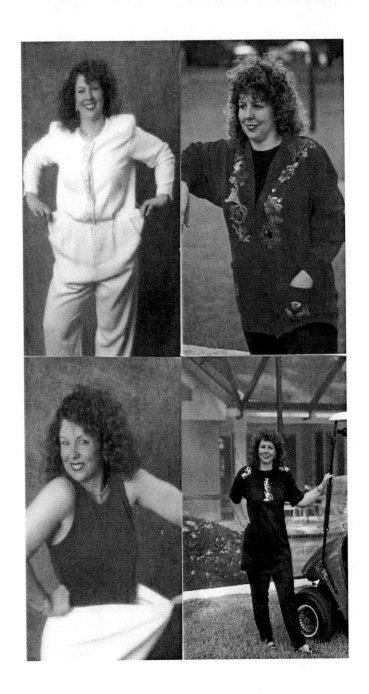

THE MOVE TO FLORIDA - I FINALLY FOUND HOME ! CHAPTER 8

Oh Yea...Welcome to the Sunshine state ! That sunshine felt so good ! I loved waking up to a blue sky and warm weather everyday, especially after the wet, cold summer that North Carolina just had. The tough part of this move was that my moving company did a horrible job in packing and moving my stuff, so almost every box had broken or damaged items in it. *It was horrible !* I cried a good bit over it. While unpacking, I realized I didn't want to travel anymore as much as I had in the summer, for two reasons. I was physically tired and Raffaella had lost a tremendous amount of weight while I was on the road and almost died. I couldn't imagine my life without her; she was all I had ! So I decide to continue my education and *finish this degree once and for all !!* I started calling the various colleges in the area and making appointments to see their campus and curriculum. I phoned one school called *Florida Metropolitan University*, a private college, and made an appointment for the next day. The lady I talked to was very sweet and polite and we ended up being good friends. This school was on the quarter system, not the semester system, and their *next quarter started on Monday. This was Friday ! I decided there was no time like the present, and what else did I have to do right then, so I enrolled.*

This being my **36th move**, I was quite used to the routine of how to get set-up and established in a new town in record time. I had already found the health food store, the massage gal, the chiropractor, and my favorite Italian restaurant. My massage lady noticed how much lactic acid had built-up in my shoulder from the worker's compensation injury and sugges - ted I drink a juice to help it. I agreed, without knowing anything about it. It was called *Noni Juice*. I was drinking 3 ounces a day for just a couple days, when I noticed my left arm was moving more freely. Within the week I could lift it over my head, something I hadn't done in over 1 ½ years. I was sold on this juice, so I joined the company in order to buy it cheaper.

I ended this year with a bang, literally ! Just 6 weeks after moving in, I had a car accident and got whiplash. Luckily I had already found a good chiro - practor and proceeded to get treatment from him. I continued to drink the *Noni Juice* and even take baths in it, as it seemed to ease the muscle spasms a lot. I was back to pre-accident status in less than 3 weeks. Both the doctor and I were shocked and amazed !

Just as I was starting to feel better, I got hit with some *even more bad news !!* I was told *I had Uterine Cancer with 6 - 12 months to live, the Monday after Thanks - giving that year. I was dumbfounded, mad, angry, hurt and scared, all wrapped up in one !!* I knew I was not going to go the traditional route, as my *"adopted mom"* had gone. She had three separate surgeries for hers, and each time it came back, until the last; she is currently 5 years cancer-free ! I had always said, *"If I got cancer, I would take care of it naturally."* Well my turn had come and now the eyes of many were upon me to see how I would react to the news.

Would I stand strong and fight it naturally or would I give in and succumb to the traditional cut, snip and tuck procedures ? Well the decision was pretty straightforward for me, as I had promised God that I would not cut on my body again after brain surgery until I was ready to come "home." So I had no choice but to do it naturally.

I decided not to tell many people, as I didn't want to start a pity-party and have people call me daily and worry over me. I shut my clothing business down to do only special orders, as I needed to focus on fighting this cancer and staying alive.

That Christmas, I made the choice not to go home, as I wanted my last Christmas to be one of peace and harmony. I knew if I went home I would have to deal with the family politics and my brother's alcoholic issues, which I had no tolerance or understanding for. Unfortunately, my angels had different plans for me. On the night of December 23rd, I was awakened from my sleep with a very vivid dream that someone had broken into my car. I decided to go down the stairs and make sure everything was ok and that this was really only a bad nightmare. *Well, my car was fine !*

As I re-entered my house, my angels (all seven of them), appeared and pro - ceeded to tell me if I didn't go home for Christmas and be civil that it would be **MY LAST ONE !!** *Well, I know my angels well enough to know they meant business, so I agreed to go.* Upon rising the next morning, I packed my bags and headed north to go home for Christmas. My parents were ecstatic to see me, and told me that it wasn't going to be a real Christ - mas without me there. *Unfortunately, I was very depressed and detached. The gifts didn't seem special to me; nothing made me smile.* I asked my mom to return all my gifts, as they were not of value to me, since I was only going to die. I asked her to just give me the money so I could return to California to see my healing family. She agreed, realizing I was only going to take care of my cancer naturally. Also, I wanted to go because they were the same people who had brought me back from *"the nearly dead"* moment back in 1996. My parents asked what I was going to do about the cancer. I said **"NOTHING !!"** I said, **"I don't believe it, first and foremost, but if I go to California and my healers tell me it is real, then I will deal with it; then and only then !!"**

I had finally reached size 4 New Years Eve 1999, and felt excited to finally get the weight off! I went to California between the quarter breaks at college in January. As I arrived, I tried to stay positive and believe the cancer was really just a scare tactic to get me moving, and was not really a disease. As I laid on the healing table listening to my healing friends channel the information to me from the masters above, I was shocked and over-whelmed with what they had to say.

They told me *"THE CANCER WAS REAL, and that I HAD CREATED IT! Me - all by myself!! All that anger, frustration, and rage that I had held inside me over all these years of recovery - had finally made it's home in my uterus (my solar plexus) and created a dis-ease called CANCER !!"*

My mind raced with the questions, "Now what? What were my options? What were my choices? How long did I have?" All these questions and many more came pouring out of my mouth. The masters continued to speak and explain to me I was an *old-soul, one of the oldest on the planet right now,* and *"we old souls"* create complex lives for ourselves down here to keep up our interests.

They told me "*I could learn to for - give, forget and let go COMPLETELY and I could cure myself of this dis-ease or I could roll-over, get human, and get scared and I would be coming home 6 months to the Day !!*" They also said if I chose to forgive and forget, they could tell me I would have three of the most fabulous years of my life afterwards. They said, *"I can't imagine, you....Acaysha, wanting to miss being the star of your own show !"* They were right about that, *but I was still scared !!* They gave me some meditation practices to do daily, told me to keep drinking *Noni juice* and in my own words of philosophy, to *start living every day to the fullest; to live it like it was my first and last day on the planet; to live it with gusto and then let go when I retired at night, starting each day anew !* It didn't sound that hard. I had dealt with so much in the last seven years; *I could do this... no problem !!*

Well, that was all fine and dandy, until I started passing blood clots and passing out ! Talk about a reality check ! I was trying to be spiritual and optimistic about this and then I got *REAL HUMAN SIGNS !* I was so scared; more scared than I had ever been in all the years previously. Unfortunately my parents didn't want to believe it or deal with it so I was left to fight this on my own. Everytime I spoke to them, I was *so mad, angry and pissed off,* that we would end up in a screaming match and one of us would hang up on the other.

I hated this ! I cried out, "*I just wanted a better life Lord. One that I could enjoy and be healthy and happy. Is that too much to ask for ?*" *Obviously it was !!*

I was really starting to see the symptoms appear in late February 2000, when I returned home from taking my midterms and passed out on my family room floor, just missing my glass table by inches. I finally was so scared, I called 911 and had the ambulance come get me. After being in the hospital for 6 hours, with no relief, and no medications, since I was allergic to the good stuff, I was simply released, only to find myself without any money or ID on me. I was able to catch a bus for most of the way as the bus driver gave me a break, and then I walked the rest of the way home !

Now I was not only in pain, and scared and alone, but I was extremely angry at the lack of family support I was getting on this. This additional anger was not helping anything; it only made things worse. I then developed a migraine headache again....this one lasted *58 straight days* ‼ It felt like I had a jackhammer on my head 24 hours a day. I finally dropped out of school, as I was scared to even drive. *Now I was mad at myself for quitting before I finished.*

On April fools day that year I called my parents in desperation and told them to come down here in the next week and get Raffaella as I was "*checking out*" of this world, meaning I was attempting suicide, for good this time ! Unfortunately, I had attempted this many times before in the last seven years so I even knew how to do it. They teach that to you in the psychiatric wards ! As usual, my mom tried to plead with me not to go, but I wasn't listening. I was worn out, not feeling loved, frustra - ted, and I wanted to quit ! This new life was way too hard for even this lady to handle. ***"Just come get me Lord !!"*** I yelled.

After several hours of talking, most of it which I was oblivious to since I had already been popping pills and drinking a large quantity of alcohol, my parents de - cided to come down and help me. It's always a sad situation when it takes major life threats like dying and suicide to get my parents' attention. They showed up the next day and I was 3/4 out of body, due to the drug overdose and alcohol content I had ingested. They were pissy with me and lacked compassion, as usual. They just proceeded to lecture me about the way I was living; my lack of exercise and my decision to live so far away from family. They tried to convince me to move closer to them saying, *"life would be better if you were closer."* *(Yea right, I wasn't buying it this time !)*

After staying a day, they took me to a Holistic show where I met a wonderful lady who worked for an innovative colour therapy company, called **Colour Energy**. This company had designed a new machine that could scan your body and tell you about your current health conditions. *I was fascinated, so I let her do mine, only to be told the cancer was alive and kicking inside of me !! I felt discouraged,* *as I thought I had made some healing progress.*

After that, my parents had the upper hand with me and proceeded to take Raffaella and I back home to South Carolina with them. My mom wanted to take me to some local medical facility, but I didn't want to go. They were already supporting the doctor's decisions to *cut, snip, tuck, zap, and kill me in the process,* without any regard to my feelings or preferences.

I was so weak and worn out and in despair that I almost fell for it, but I was saved by the grace of God !! I decided to go lay down and take a nap, and while asleep, in my dreams, *God spoke to me.*

God said, "my child, we had a deal; you promised me you would not cut on your body until you are ready to come home. I gave you grace once, a year after surgery, but I will not give you grace this time." "You have

the power within you to cure this.
Are you going to stand strong and do
it the right way or succumb to the
human easy way out and come home
my child." "The decision is yours, but
I stand by our original deal."

I woke up almost in a panic, yet feeling relieved at the same time. I told only my mom about the experience, as my father is not a believer. My mom, knowing I was going to do what I thought was best, no matter what they thought or felt, decided to let me go home and deal with it in my way. Unfortunately, I left with a bad taste in my mouth, as they said *"if I didn't move home and do it their way, then I was on my own to deal with this, as they were TOO BUSY socially to be bothered with me living 600 miles away !"* *So be it !! I didn't like to break my promises I made to GOD anyway !!*

So I got on a plane and returned home, leaving Raffaella with my parents, just in case I decided to go home and kill myself. I wasn't home 6 days when I was missing Raffaella so badly I could hardly bare it. She was my best friend; my healer and my angel, so I decided to drive back up there and get her. I was there only 3 hours when we got into another heated discussion. Exhausted, I took a quick nap and then got back on the road to return to Florida, my home state !

The next three weeks were horrible, as the migraines were quite intense and I just felt beat-up in more ways than one. *All alone, with no family support or love, I was in this battle and had to fight it by myself !! (Like I had done for the last seven years !) Me, the angels, and GOD... with them by my side, I knew I could do it !!* On that Thursday night going into Easter weekend, I went into prayer to give my resignation notice to the Lord. I do lots of work for the Lord down here on this planet and I help a lot of people. I'm a great friend to many, and a healer to others, and I told God I wanted to quit if he/she couldn't help me get well. I told God that I wasn't going to work for him/her in any capacity anymore without being healthy. I told God I wasn't going to heal another person down here and that I was going to kill myself over the Easter weekend ! I figured as long as people would be celebrating the death and resurrection of Christ on that weekend, that they could celebrate my death and my return to heaven too !! *I was very truthful and very honest explaining that I was tired, frustrated, all alone and beaten-up too much to keep enduring this pain.* I had been living with and enduring these migraine headaches now for *58 straight days*, and it felt like a constant jack - hammer on my head.

After that long and detailed talk with God, I drank a couple bottles of wine, and rolled over on the couch and went to sleep. I woke the next morning feeling very unattached to my body, only to realize I didn't have a migraine headache and I didn't hurt anywhere ! I felt like I was out-of-body; like between two worlds most of the day and *without a migraine headache too !!* I later realized I had received a healing during the night and now I was floating above my body. *I guess God was listening that night and valued my work down here on earth...Thank You God !!*

 That Easter weekend was a _huge turning point in my life. I had received a healing, was cured of cancer and migraine headaches, and also met my soul mate on my computer that week – end !!_ I began to chat online with a wonderful young man, who turned my life completely around for the better. He was *my angel in disguise* and a much needed one at that ! He was an answer to a very long-standing prayer that I have prayed for, for so many, many years. *"Mr. Casa – nova"* came into my life at a time when I had given up; when I saw no hope or reason to continue to live. He brought laughter and love into my life, and gave me the courage to finish my college degree. He allowed me to grow and learn what *"real love"* was about !

Move over Cinderella, I've got you beat !!

I was so in love and living life to the fullest; I thanked God everyday !

Those masters were right; the next three years were going to be fabulous! FINALLY, I actually got to find out what <u>real true love</u> was all about. There wasn't a romance novel on the market as good as this was. He was a pilot and would fly in to see me. *It was so exciting, passionate and erotic ! He taught me how to love to the deepest levels; levels I didn't know existed ! I felt so alive, and so happy !!* I had finally found peace, and a security within me, something I had never felt this lifetime, especially around men ! Just having him in the same area as me, he made me feel so complete and loved. I felt so blessed to be alive again ! He taught me to laugh, love and be young at heart.

During the summer, I returned to California to settle all of my worker's compensation lawsuits, and I won them all ! While out there, I decided to make an appointment to see my gynecologist who used to treat me and had him check on my cancer status for me. *The test results came back a month later and there was **NO CANCER IN MY BODY !!** I was so relieved and ecstatic*; I made my sweetheart a candlelight dinner he will never forget so we could celebrate the great news.

This relationship taught me so much about life and myself in general. He didn't buy me flowers, candy or cards, but he didn't have to. Our love was so true and complete, I knew he loved me, without anything written or bought. Our passion was so intense and deep that I would drive 1 1/2 hours to go see him in the middle of the night, just to make hot passionate love with him, and then turn around and return home the next morning. *I didn't care about the lack of sleep; it was so exciting, real and erotic I would do it again in a heart beat !!*

We got to live moments and fan - tasies that other people only imagine or dream about...we did them. We made love in the swimming pool, in the hot tub, on the beach, in the shower; you name it we did. **It was so hot, erotic and passion - ate, it felt like a dream – a dream come true !!** I finally met a guy who could satisfy all of my needs and make me feel so much like a real lady and a queen in her own palace ! We even went on a cruise to the Bahamas to celebrate the completion of my college bachelor's degree in October 2000. *Oh what a very different and passionate "surgery anniversary" that year was !!* **Eight years seizure free** *and it was only getting better !*

Life couldn't be more perfect. I thought, maybe this *"soul-mate"* idea is real and I have finally found mine !

This relationship made me look at all the others in the past, and made me realize how superficial they were ! How I used to only get flowers and cards when we had fights because the guy was trying to make up with me. They would do this only so they would have a date for the weekend, not because they truly loved me !

During this time I wrote many poems about our love, my dreams and my passions. I will share them with you in the next chapter of this book. *We shared many deep moments and memories to - gether, ones that no one can replace !* I have had many dreams of the future we will share and my poems will express those to you. *I hope too that you have found your soul mate and are living the life you are destined to live on this planet.*

A COLLECTION OF POEMS WRITTEN BY ME ABOUT LOVE AND LIFE

CHAPTER 9

FOR THE MAN I WANT TO SPEND THE REST OF MY LIFE WITH....

You are my love and my life,

You understand all my thoughts and share in all my dreams.

You understand and support whatever I do and I never thought your support could make such a difference, that your encouragement would bring my dreams closer, make my successes sweeter and my losses easier to accept.

I LOVE YOU

For being so honest and trustworthy,

For being so fun and exciting,

For being strong, yet so gentle and sensitive,

For being such an outstanding person,

I LOVE YOU

For all you do for me,

For all you express to me,
For all you share with me,
And for all that you are.

I never suspected that we would discover so many common interests and values, or that I could ever enjoy simple pleasures as much as when they are shared with you.
I had no idea how easy you would be to talk to, to trust and to share my deepest secrets and feelings with.

You are the one person that I trust my life with and whom I always want to be with.
You are My Love.

I never imagined that I would grow to want, to need and to love you so much.
When you first came into my life, I never dreamed you'd soon be someone I couldn't live without.

I LOVE YOU

OUR LOVE IS STRONGER BECAUSE OF ALL THAT WE'VE BEEN THROUGH TOGETHER...

Relationships are never easy, and you and I have had our share of struggling and troubled times, but together we made it.

Together, we cared enough to face our problems - we loved enough not to let go.

And now, what we have is even stronger because of all we've been through, and all we struggled with.

I sometimes worry about the future, but with you by my side, the future seems much brighter - the present more precious, more meaningful.

We need the tears to appreciate the laughter.

We must share our problems to realize how much we truly need each other, to give our love the chance to expand, to strengthen, to endure.

We deserve nothing less than a love that will remain through all aspects of our lives.

Together, we will face all obstacles with confidence, because we already know our relationship can endure even the worst of times,

As long as we love - share and stay together !

YOU ARE EVERYTHING I EVER
DREAMED LOVE COULD BE

You are my love.
You are the person who holds me when I need to be held.
You are the person I share my everyday thoughts and concerns with, the one who understands and comforts me.
You are my bright tomorrow.

I want to be all of those things to you.
I want to be able to give you all the love you need.
And also the time you need to develop your own interests and reach your own goals.

We have made a commitment to love and respect one another, and I want you to know that my commitment to you is still strong and true.
My love for you is still growing deeper,
And my heartfelt wish for you is to have the best that life can offer, ALWAYS !

YOUR LOVE MEANS SO MUCH TO ME

Love is a special word, rich with meaning,
Overflowing in thought.
Love is sharing - sharing happiness and sorrow, the blue
skies and gray, the important and everyday concerns of
life.
Love is understanding - a quiet understanding in which a
thought may not be spoken but is understood.
Above all, love is sharing everything, together.

The many hopes and plans we share,
The joys we're dreaming of have brought new meaning to
my life.
Since I have had you to love....
And as I wish you happiness, today and all year through,
I want to say how much it means to have your love and
you.

LIFE'S TWISTS AND TURNS

Life is full of twists and turns; no one said it was going to be easy, straight and narrow with no bends, bumps or curves in the road.

Life really is one lifelong "test" of one's faith; how much you believe, how much you withstand, how far you'll bend, and where is your breaking point ?

Everyone's breaking point is at a different level and only God really knows where it is, as He / She is always pushing on it and pushing it higher and higher. The tough times can be very trying, stressful and emotionally draining, but when the experience is over you are wiser and stronger and with more faith than before.

Life really is just a series of short plays, each with a different set of actors or actresses, each with a new and different theme and outcome each and every time.

So stop taking life so seriously and learn to enjoy the ride. Realize you are the star of your own play, so lighten up, laugh more and live it to the fullest.

Life is definitely a play, except there are no rehearsals, as it changes every day. When one gets too lax or comfortable, life delivers a new challenge to unpack.

Unfortunately most challenges don't come with instruction manuals or guides !

When one thinks life is so bad with no hope for the future, God will bring in an angel to lift you up and give you new energy and hope.

Sometimes these angels will stay a long time; others will disappear in the middle of the night. Some will back off to give you space to grow and experience new things.

They move far enough away that you miss them more, but are still close enough for you to know they are near.

Absence makes the heart grow fonder and truer, and you learn to appreciate those in your life more.

WHEN TWO PEOPLE FALL IN LOVE...

When two people fall in love, they share equally with each other.

They become one.

A bond is built, along with trust and loyalty.

They accept each other for what they are.

They love each other for who they are.

They are there for each other, to comfort when they are down.

When one hurts, the other hurts.

They communicate with each other.

The problems they have are worked out.

They work on their relationship together.

They learn to grow with each other.

They accept challenges as they come.

Sometimes they are scared, but they are always there for one another.

They are one, but they have their own minds, their own ideas and different ways of thinking.

They love and learn, cry and feel.

They are there to help each other.

They are not perfect; they make mistakes.

Their lives are lived happily, when two people fall in love.

LOVE IS....

Something no one can really explain.

It's a feeling, a warmth, an inner peace.

Sometimes it feels like a warm bear hug.

Sometimes it feels like butterflies in your tummy.

Sometimes its feels like an overload or surge of energy,

And sometimes it is a quiet inner peace.

Real true love is hard to find,

And even harder to let go or lose.

Love can make your world worth living,

And it can rob you of all you value.

Love can bring new light and wisdom to an old situation
or problem,

But when lost it can create a whole new set of scenarios.

To truly give one's heart and soul to another is a scary
and risky move,

As the outcome is unpredictable.

One may take it, nurture and love it, allowing you to grow, and in return share theirs with you, a total moment or lifetime of love.

One may only take and not share, and use it for their pleasure and gain, leaving it by the wayside when they see fit and have no more use of it.

Love is so simple, yet so complex.
Love is so pure and gentle, until it has been used and abused.
Love completes a person.

Once hurt, one has a hard time ever giving of themself totally to another; the walls and barriers go up and can become almost impossible to break down.

Love can give one hopes and dreams they never thought was possible or attainable in one lifetime,

But when lost it can rob them of everything of value and importance.

Love is a crazy thing.... You can't live with it,
but you can't live without it either !!

MY FUTURE AND DREAMS,
"THE CENTER" CHAPTER 10

My first career goal has been completed, as you are reading my first book, hopefully one of many to come ! I am hoping to help others move through their challenges and difficulties that they face in this lifetime, and to inspire more epileptics to step out of the comfort zone and have the miraculous surgery that can help them to start living their lives ! *My book is meant to be an inspiration to everyone, whether you are fighting a major illness or dis-ease or you are just having a bad day. This book is meant to inspire and motivate you by giving you the strength to keep going and find new answers and hope for your own life.* We are all here for a reason, some of us know what it is, the rest of us walk around looking for it, and always wondering ! What's your purpose ?

My ultimate professional goal is to become a professional speaker, (the female Zig Ziglar of the world), a healer and an inspiration to many. Not only for epileptics, but also for anyone trying to overcome an illness or disability, even just those feeling discouraged or depressed. I feel like I can conquer anything now with no limitations....

"The sky is not even my limit !!"

Through this great journey of all the stages of recovery and my new life, I have seen *the blackest of days, the brightest of dawns, the scariest moments, the greatest despair and the best of achieve - ments and accomplishments one could ever experience.* I am now equipped to better handle life and its challenges and have now learned how to never give up, no matter how tough and trying it may get. I have become very spiritual and holistic; learning natural ways to heal and feel good. Little did I know how much this experience would benefit me personally and career wise in the future. I believe any goal I set is worth achieving, no matter how many obstacles I have to overcome !

"I hope to inspire you, motivate you and delight you, leaving you counting your blessings !!"

I plan to share my newfound wisdom and life experiences with the general public as my wonderful team of angels continue to teach me new ways of living, loving and laughing.

"My angels have taught me so much about life, love, and laughter, and how to really enjoy the journey we are all on, and now I am being guided to share that knowledge with you ! "

My other futuristic dream is to build an *all-inclusive holistic center* for people to come to; one center where they will be able to find natural answers to their health problems. As I walked along my path to this new life, I searched the world over, looking for great masters, healers and teachers that would teach me and show

me new ways to get well, naturally ! I was
even willing to move closer to one, if I
thought they could help me get well !
*I spent many hours seeking these people
out, and now realize that most people
don't have the time, patience or endurance
to do this much research !* So I would like
to bring the best of each holistic and
natural field practitioner to one place.

Medicine has it's place in society
and I thank them for the technology of my
surgery, but I do believe GOD didn't make
junk and we don't need *all those drugs
and surgeries !* I think we can heal and
cure our bodies naturally, if we just have
the resources and tools available to us. So
my dream is to bring the best of all natural
practitioners to you in one facility located
in Florida.

There you would be able to get a
massage, a chiropractic adjustment, an
acupuncture treatment, a reflexology
treatment, rolfing, cranial sacral work, and
many others types of natural treatments to

help enhance your total body, all which I have experienced personally along my path to healing. Not to mention, a psychic reading, numerology reading, astrology charts, colour therapy and many, many more alternative treatments ! I also want to have a bookstore and chapel on the grounds, so you can read and find answers to your own life's issues. To be able to have quiet time either in the chapel or on the grounds, just being with nature and God !

I want to help empower the people of today and make a difference in their lives tomorrow. So as you can see, I have big dreams and goals for this lifetime ! If you are interested in knowing more about the Holistic Center I want to build or want to help me build it, please contact me.

ACAYSHA (772) 336 -8322

or email me at

acaysha@newhorizonsandmyangels.com

THE CONCLUSION - CHAPTER 11

So in conclusion, I have lived a very diverse and adventuresome life, one many people envy. I have moved and lived all over the world, 38 times ! I did 11 of them before the age of 21! I am a motivated, optimistic, go-getter, and have always taken on any challenge life has given me. I was raised to be a fighter –*THANKS MOM !* As you have now found out, I am a very complex, detailed lady who is on her second life in the same body....

EPILEPSY AND CANCER FREE !!

I hope my book has helped you, inspired you, or given you a new hope to move through your challenges and diffi - culties you face in this lifetime. Whether you are fighting a major illness or dis-ease, or you are just having a bad day; *this book is meant to inspire and motivate you by giving you the strength to keep going and find new answers and hope for your own life.*

I hope I have inspired more epilep -
tics to step out of their comfort zone and
have the surgery and start living their lives
more completely ! Many epileptics are
labeled handicapped; because people are
scared of the attacks, but under that scary
surface is usually a wonderful person,
waiting to emerge !

Through all stages of my recovery
and journey into my new life; I have now
learned how to persevere and never give
up, no matter how tough and trying it may
get ! *I believe any goal I set is worth
achieving, no matter how many obstacles I
have to overcome !* Obstacles became my
middle name for a while, because I was re-
learning every aspect and phase of life.

I am now better equipped to handle
life and its challenges. I have tried many
ways and techniques; not all were easy and
stress free. Through this *"boot camp"*
training of life over these last ten years;
consisting of growing up, learning to cook
again, finding myself, working, playing,

discovering balance and just under -
standing the game of life, I have now
blossomed into a wonderful dynamic
young lady, who knows who she is and
where she is going.

Nothing is going to stop me now !!

This has been the hardest, most
challenging, exciting, invigorating, and
frustrating thing I have ever undertaken
before in this lifetime, but IT WAS
WORTH IT !!!

Thanks Dr. Zimmerman and Dr.
Hirschorn for making this possible !!
THANKS MOM and DAD for everything,
no matter how much I struggled, I still
love you !! I hope we can all heal and
move forward from this moment on, as I
want to help so many people do the
same.

Here is my most current picture of me, taken at my graduation in October 2000.

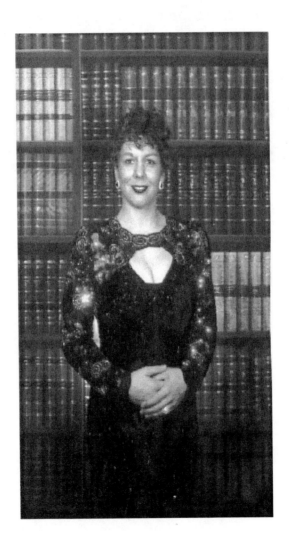

You see life is full of challenges, experiences and adventures. Every day is a new day - so take it and run with it and live it to the fullest ! I hope you enjoyed the journey down memory lane with me.

If I can help you in any way, please feel free to contact me on my websites at

www.acaysha.com

or

www.newhorizonsandmyangels.com

or email me at

acaysha@newhorizonsandmyangels.com

HAVE A BLESSED AND WONDERFUL LIFE !!!

GOD BLESS YOU !!

ISBN 1553694597-7